Common Sense Health

A Guide for Preventing and Reversing Lifestyle Diseases

By Feng-Ling Wang

Bambridge Medical Arts, Inc.
Boise, Idaho Printed in the USA

Common Sense Health A Guide for Preventing and Reversing Lifestyle Diseases

First American Edition

Printed in the United States of America

Library of Congress Cataloging-in-Publication Data

Wang, Feng-Ling
Common sense health : a guide for preventing and reversing lifestyle diseases / Feng-Ling Wang.
p.   cm.
Includes bibliographical references.
ISBN 978-159216-013-6
1. Prevention of Disease 2. Promotion of Health 3. Medical Care 4. Health Care
2012912727

ISBN 978-1-59216-013-6
LCCN 2012912727

Visit www.bambridgemedicalarts.com

Important Notice and Disclaimer

Contents

Chapter One

Modern Medicine
Meets
Common Sense

I was born and raised in a rural area of central China. I grew up in a culture that had remained unchanged for centuries. Tractors and bicycles were the most advanced machines I was exposed to for the majority of my childhood. Almost everything we needed was produced by hand. Even the clothes and shoes my family wore were hand sewn by my mother and grandmother. Throughout primary school and middle school I walked a total of ten miles to and from my home to school every school day. We didn't have electricity in our homes, which meant there was no television, so kids created and played games together for entertainment. After school, kids would help their parents with the necessary farm work. Life was very simple.

My diet was naturally organic and healthy. We ate what we grew. Often this was the only food we had. The bulk of my diet consisted of whole grains such as wheat, corn, sweat potatoes, soy beans and vegetables. I rarely ate meat or eggs. Eating meat was reserved for special occasions. We were able to eat meat or eggs about once per month.

Because we didn't have electricity, my sleep schedule was determined by the sunrise and sunset. I went to sleep when the sun set and woke up before the sun rose. Everyone was used to the temperature inside the house being the same temperature as the temperature outdoors. I never even dreamt about having an air conditioner or heater.

Medical doctors were not available, but medications did not need to be prescribed by a doctor because people were expected to use their best judgment to choose the right medicine (such as antibiotics). Only when people fell seriously ill would they go to the city to receive treatment from medical professionals. Barely anyone was overweight. Only one person out of the town's two thousand residents had diabetes. All of the families in the area experienced similar financial conditions, coexisted peacefully and were generally happy with their lives.

The environment was natural and free from chemicals. We had no chemicals in our home, not even cleaning products. The only chemicals used were pesticides in the cotton fields. When people came to visit the country from the city, it was easy to smell the chemical rich scents of the shampoos, conditioners, lotions and perfumes they used. The main sources of environmental and air pollution came from burning straw or wood used to cook meals. The air was fresh and the sky was blue, so as a boy I often spent time lying down in nature and looking up at the sky.

My mom's family was well known throughout the area for doing acupuncture and herbal medicine. Whenever I got sick or had any sort of ailment my grandmother treated me with natural medicine and acupressure. I spent much of my free time in the clinic watching my grandparents treat their patients. They would always tell me little health habit tips and explain to me why they would choose different types of herbs and acupuncture points for different ailments. I remember hearing two pieces of advice frequently. I was told that if I ate heated liquids and foods that my chance of getting a stomach ache would be reduced and if I dressed warm I would be less likely to catch a cold. Even today those are the two most popular pieces of health advice in China. The status of my health throughout my life is proof that listening to this kind of common sense can prevent health problems. There are so many examples of these types of simple, common sense tips that can truly impact the quality of your health on a daily basis.

The community, concerned with taking care of each other's well-being, would share health wisdom with each other. This collection of practical wisdom became ingrained in our culture as we adjusted our way of life and accepted personal responsibility for our health. Well known advice included, "Spicy or dry food can scratch your throat. A scratched throat easily becomes a sore throat." "Keep yourself warm to prevent and treat joint pain." "Eating too much fruit can rot your teeth, so always drink water after you eat sweet foods." Observing this knowledge and following the advice helped me maintain good health. I not only experienced the benefits of using this advice to maintain my health, but I became so interested in how health problems can be prevented that I was inspired to go to medical school and pursue a career in acupuncture and alternative medicine.

I was fourteen years old the first time I experienced stress and pressure. My family had just acquired basic electricity and, for the first time, we had lighting in our home. I began to read books, newspapers and magazines and started to learn about city life. I developed the desire to move out of the country and into the city. I knew that I needed to study hard in order to meet the qualifications to become a college candidate. College education is free in China, but it is very competitive because there are many more students applying for entrance than there are college openings available. At the time I applied to attend college only ten percent of high school students were accepted into all universities in China. Few high school teachers in the countryside had degrees; most had barely even graduated from high school. (When I was a child, China was still recovering from the Cultural Revolution which had caused the country's school system to severely suffer.) I had to study on my own so that I would be able to compete with students from the cities who would be testing to be awarded the few college entrances available. The students from the cities had the advantages of better schools and access to more resources, such as libraries and tutors; things that simply were not available to me in the countryside. The high level of stress that I experienced during this time temporarily depressed me, but after a while it taught me how to handle stress and it built my tolerance to stress.

Working hard and studying on my own got me accepted and enrolled into Beijing University of Chinese Medicine. The stress and pressure that I experienced in high school was never surpassed, not even in college, where I had an intense workload studying both Eastern and Western medical knowledge in a five year time frame. The stress of college caused by the intense workload led to several of my classmates (many who had been from the city and did not have to struggle to gain their spots in college) to not be able to physically or emotionally handle these pressures. They had less common knowledge about how to care for their physical and mental health because they hadn't grown up in a community so concerned with personal responsibility for self as I had. The students from the city had been trained to go to a clinic when they didn't feel good. They hadn't learned how to care for themselves with prevention or how to rely on the folk wisdom of their culture. Many of them developed health problems because of it.

I was always convinced that I wanted to study alternative medicine and have always been a serious advocate of preventative medicine, but when I went to college my friends and family tried to convince me to specialize in western medicine and surgery. When I started college I had six roommates. All of us had intended to specialize in acupuncture. Four of my roommates switched their majors to orthopedic surgery. Out of my graduating class of eighty physicians, fifty-four became orthopedic surgeons. In all, twenty-six of my classmates specialized in acupuncture and out of those, only five (including myself) actually work as acupuncturists today. After I graduated and completed my residency in 1996, I always used acupuncture, acupressure and herbs as my main modes of treatment. I only prescribed Western pharmaceuticals or recommended surgery for my patients on very rare occasions.

When I moved to the United States in 1997, I slowly became acquainted with the Western way of life. The culture and lifestyle were new to me. Before I came to America, I had read that the American food industry had some of the best regulations, standards and food sources in the world; therefore, I assumed that American food was safe (and healthy) to consume. I read about how much Americans loved to exercise, which explained why Americans always won the most gold medals at the Olympics. I knew that the United States was world famous for their medical advances and treatment options. I had read and heard so many positive things about America's health standards and healthcare system. But, after living and practicing Chinese medicine in America for fifteen years, I have gained a lot of experience and learned that there are many serious problems with the American lifestyle and America's approach to health. In my practice, I strive to emphasize to each one of my patients to focus on their own ability to recover from and avoid illness through preventative care. The more I observed the American lifestyle and diseases common to it, the more I saw how great of a role preventative health could play in solving the American health crisis. And yes, America is currently in a severe health crisis.

First and foremost, America's approach to food and eating habits needs to be drastically altered. For example, toxic (highly carcinogenic) food preparation techniques such as frying, grilling and smoking have become the main types of cooking styles in America. Many people are puzzled and deceived by various health articles, such as articles that claim you should eat as much meat as possible for protein, that there is too much arsenic in rice or that soybeans have high allergen rates. These types of articles have inspired a lot of fear and confusion in the American people and have led to a lot of faulty logic and decisions with regards to making dietary choices. In this book I will be discussing some common sense health concepts that the American public at large has lost touch with and, perhaps, has never had the opportunity to learn. I will be discussing various aspects of what makes a healthy diet, including how preparing, cooking and storing food can impact your health.

The second most important thing I have observed about America's view of health is the emphasis that has been placed on sports rather than exercise. It is important to understand that sports and exercise are not the same things. Exercise is mainly designed for health purposes, whereas sports are designed for entertainment, not necessarily health purposes. If not done properly, both exercise and sports can damage your health rather than preserve or improve it. In America, improper exercise and sports activities are a major cause of body pain and injury. People forget to take into account various factors when exercising such as their career, age, health status, etc. This book will help present and explain some of the factors you should consider when developing an exercise routine, as well as help you to find which sports are best suited to your individual needs.

Many people come from broken homes, have to deal with emotionally charged pasts and are generally very emotionally turbulent. Many people treat their emotional problems with medication, but it is important to understand that all people experience emotional ups and downs throughout life. It is very important to learn skills that will help you regulate your emotions. This book will give you tools to help manage stress, emotions and your mind (such as determination and self-discipline). Additionally, this book will explain the intimate relationship between sleep quality and mental health, which is a relationship that is not commonly understood in America.

Turning to medication and surgery to solve health problems is the standard of American health care. When you look at global statistics of life expectancy, quality of life, general well-being, access to appropriate health care, etc. you start to see that Americans do not have the greatest health care system or the highest standard (quality) of living in the world; in fact, America is quickly losing ground to the rest of the developed world in all of these areas.[1] A significant percentage of the American population takes unnecessary medication, simply because they do not know how to prevent illness or seek proper treatment. Many of them are too afraid to even discuss alternative treatment options with their doctors. (By this, I mean alternatives to prescription medications or surgery.) Taking unnecessary medication can actually cause your health to deteriorate, can diminish your quality of life and shorten your lifetime. This book will help you become an informed patient, so that when you collaborate with your doctor, your chances of taking unnecessary medication and having unnecessary surgery will significantly decrease.

Tobacco, drug (including illegal and legal drugs—especially opiates) and alcohol abuse are huge problems in America. Most people are not fully aware of the extreme physical and emotional costs of drug and alcohol misuse and abuse. This book will help you to understand the serious health damage that can result from drug and alcohol abuse and will, hopefully, give you the willpower to discipline yourself to be able to cut down or quit these altogether.

The use of chemically based products is deeply interwoven into the average American's lifestyle. Most people would rather smell chemicals than natural odors. People often talk about external environmental pollution, but most people do not realize how much chemical pollution is in their own homes (perfumes, air sprays, cleaning products, cooking pollution, etc.). This book will help you to identify carcinogenic scents in order to rid your home of them and help you avoid breathing in toxic chemicals.

Driving is the main mode of transportation for most Americans. Unfortunately, if you drive, it is almost inevitable that you will be involved in a car crash at some point in your lifetime. Vehicle collisions can cause debilitating health conditions and seriously worsen the quality of your life. The chapter on avoiding automobile collisions will give you important and useful information on how to effectively decrease your chances of getting into a car crash.

Overall, this book provides you with an introduction to crucial, yet common, concepts and actions that you can use to understand how to take care of and preserve your health starting today. This book will provide you with a detailed explanation of why it is so important to place the responsibility of your health in your own hands. The information I present in this book is relatively easy to understand. I use common language and avoid technical terminology in my explanation of key points. You do not need a medical degree to understand the topics discussed in this book. If you take the time to understand these concepts and integrate what you learn into your lifestyle, you can save time, money and improve the quality of your life. These common sense concepts are, I believe, the answers to America's health crisis. The information in this book will help you to open your mind to new ideas and different ways of approaching health and proper care of the human body. I want you to realize that good health is not synonymous with your access to and use of health insurance, doctors or prescription medications. Rather, it is my goal to help you learn that good health is up to you and the lifestyle choices you make. Pursuing good health can change your life, the life of your family, friends and ultimately, society as a whole.

Chapter Two

Why Most Diseases Are Food-caused and What You Can Do About It

Most people claim to know how to eat, but the truth is that the majority of illnesses and diseases are related to what we eat. With so much information about which diets are best, coming from so many different sources, it is easy to become confused about what is the best way to eat for your health. You may even feel so overwhelmed from so much conflicting information on the market today that you don't even know where to start or how to plan a healthy diet. With a little common sense knowledge however, you will be better able to make the best choices for yourself. Let's start by answering a few of the biggest, most common questions about maintaining a balanced diet today.

Big Question 1: How Many Calories Do I Really Need?

It is common to hear that the average adult needs to eat about two thousand calories per day. This, of course, is an oversimplified recommendation. Most people don't truly understand how much food they should eat in order to maintain their own personal health. This is, in fact, the most common question my patients ask me. It is difficult for a medical practitioner to answer this question because the amount each individual should eat is dependent on many factors. Not taking all individual factors into account causes people to misunderstand how many calories and which types of food they should be eating.

For example, if you eat a meal of only steamed vegetables, you may eat two or three hundred calories, but if you eat bread and beef until you are full, you may eat close to one thousand calories during one meal. The most common cause of health problems is the overconsumption of calories, not necessarily how much (volume) we eat. Each person should have a different diet and consume calories from different sources. When you ask, "How much should I eat?" You should be asking, "How many calories should I eat on a daily basis?" This question is still difficult to answer because it depends on your activity level, ideal weight and individual health conditions. Some people say that an office worker should eat about twelve hundred to eighteen hundred calories a day, but there is no way this can apply to all office workers. Here are some suggestions to help you know understand daily calorie intake.

The more physically active you are, the more calories you should consume. For example, if your job includes hard, physical labor or if you are an active, athletic person, you should eat more calories. If you are active enough, you don't need to worry about how many calories you eat, that is, it is possible to be active enough that counting calories will no longer be necessary for you. If you play competitive sports you will burn two or more times the calories you burn from a taking a casual walk over the same amount of time.

The higher your body mass, the more calories you need. For example, if you weigh seventy pounds you should definitely be eating less then somebody who weighs two-hundred pounds. How much you should eat depends on your body structure and build. If you weigh two-hundred pounds and you are a 5'1" female, you should not be eating as much as a male who is 6'2" and weighs two-hundred pounds. The taller and bigger you are, the more calories you will need to consume because your body, in general, requires more calories to perform necessary functions.

Different health conditions require different amounts of calories to be consumed. If you are overweight you will probably need to eat less than your body needs at its current weight in order to lose weight or avoid gaining weight. Overconsumption of calories is the main cause of being overweight. When I tell my overweight patients that they eat too much, many of them tell me that they do not eat much at all; some even say they only eat one meal a day. But, it is not about how much you eat, it is about how many calories you consume. That is, the type of food you eat is more important than the amount of food you eat. If you are average weight and eat only one three thousand calorie meal each day, you will still be eating more calories than you need. I had one patient who wanted to lose weight. She complained to me that she didn't eat much and couldn't understand why she wasn't losing weight. I suggested she get a book that explained how many calories were in different foods so she could use it to count how many calories she was eating. I told her to not change her diet, but to just keep track of how many calories she was consuming. When she returned to see me a couple of weeks later, she showed me her record of how many calories she had eaten. The totaled numbers showed that, on average, she was consuming almost five thousand calories per day. Even though she didn't eat that much (volume) at meals, she did snack a lot. In fact, she consumed more calories through snacking than from her actual meals. She had been choosing calorie dense foods that didn't seem like "a lot" or large portioned, but were, indeed "packed" with calories. I helped her change the types of food she was eating and she was able to reduce her daily caloric intake and achieve her weight loss goals. Losing weight cannot happen until you control how many calories you eat. If you have hyperglycemia or diabetes you have to be extra cautious about how much and what types of food you eat. In these cases, it may be best for you to consult with a professional dietician who can help you properly modify your diet.

Metabolic syndrome (a group of diseases common in wealthy nations that includes high blood pressure, hyperglycemia and high cholesterol) is caused by the overconsumption of calories. Extra calories can be turned into cholesterol in your body. Metabolic syndrome is not just caused by eating too much of certain types of food, like foods high in animal fat or sugar; it can also be caused by the overconsumption of "healthy foods" such as whole grains, olive oil or fish. Many people think that eating too much salt causes a rise in blood pressure or that eating too much sugar causes diabetes. This is, in part, true, but the main cause of high blood pressure and diabetes is the overconsumption of calories. These health problems can be controlled by seriously altering your diet (a dietician may be necessary) by eating less calories. In time, you may find that by eating the right types of food, you will be able to feel full while consuming fewer calories. For example, you may find that you are satisfied more by eating a full bowl of fresh salad greens, with relatively few calories, than you are by eating a small sized french-fry, with relatively high calories. This change will not only reduce your overall caloric intake, but will also increase the amount of nutrients you eat, such as trace minerals and vitamins that are absolutely essential for good health.

Your caloric intake requirement also depends on how well your digestive system functions. If your digestive system does not function correctly, you will not be able to break down food and absorb it; this will prevent you from utilizing all of the calories you consume. In this case, you will need to eat more in order to compensate for the wasted calories and avoid nutritional deficiency. For example, some people who have food allergies or intolerances have a harder time breaking down and digesting certain foods. Foods that you are not sensitive to are easier for your body to digest and absorb. So, depending on the foods you eat, the amount of calories you will need will be different.

Age is another factor that affects individual caloric requirements. An older person's digestive system works differently than a younger person's digestive system. Because arteriosclerosis (hardening of the veins) is common in older people, their digestive system does not function as effectively. Therefore, food cannot be broken down, absorbed and digested as well as when they were younger. An older person may take in the same amount of calories as when they were young, but due to their decreased digestive functions, their bodies may not absorb the same amount of nutrition as they did when they were young. Older people tend to lose their appetites or prefer to eat less as well. Because of this, it is important that an elderly person evaluate how much nutrition they require with their physician and make adjustments or add supplements (such as vitamins or nutritional drinks) if necessary.

If you are pregnant, you have to eat more because you are eating for two people. You need to make sure you are taking in enough nutrition for both yourself and your fetus. If you are underweight or are seriously ill, you should consume more calories than would normally be recommended for a healthy pregnant woman.

Another factor is temperature. Your body loses more body heat and burns more calories in cold temperatures and during winter, so you will need to eat more depending on the temperature.

Some foods can be easier to digest than others. For example, calories you consume from seafood are much easier to digest and break down than calories that come from whole grains. So, the types of food you eat can, in part, determine how many calories you should eat. Generally, you choose to eat fewer foods that contain easy to break down calories and consume more calories from foods that are harder to break down.

Taking all of this into consideration, I cannot suggest to you how many calories you need because the amount will depend on many factors such as your height, ideal weight, digestive health, general health and activity level. All of these factors will be different for every person on any given day. You should eat what your body needs and what is fit for your health needs. The easiest way to determine whether or not you eat enough or overeat is to track your weight. If you gain weight, then it is most likely that you are eating more calories than your body needs.

Watching your weight is the most convenient way to know whether or not you overeat. If you lose weight or cannot maintain a certain healthy weight, then you should probably eat more. This may apply to persons who are very physically active. If you are a runner and you lose weight when you increase activity, then you should add more calories to your diet. Of course, if you lose weight for no reason, you may need to see a physician to see if there is a medical reason for your unintended weight loss.

It is important to have your cholesterol checked regularly. People who have already had a stroke, heart attack or heart problem need to eat fewer calories in order to prevent having another stroke or heart attack. Consuming too many calories can cause high cholesterol, high blood pressure, high glucose levels (hyperglycemia) or diabetes.

You know yourself the best. The more you study, the more you will learn about how to treat your individual, unique body and health. Ancient Chinese medicine approaches life, health and diet as a balancing act. It is hard to know what to eat and how much to eat for every meal, but the more you try to eat a balanced, well-rounded diet, the more balanced your health will be. Remember, eat to live and do not live to eat.

Big Question 2: How Much Should I Eat?

Eat a calorically and nutritionally balanced diet and eat until comfortably full. Consuming too many vitamins and minerals can be toxic for your body. Eating too much of certain foods such as fruit, vegetables, nuts or dairy can trigger health problems for some individuals. For example, drinking too much milk may cause diarrhea for some (lactose intolerance), while eating too many vegetables can cause bloating and gas for others (sensitivity to fiber). Feeling full is satisfying; it is important for both your digestive tract and your mind. A full stomach signals digestive enzymes to continue to be produced and maintains the normal activity of the digestive tract. In our modern lifestyle, people tend to eat calorie dense foods until they are full, as opposed to low calorie foods. A bellyful of high calorie food is the number one killer of the average person's health. High calorie foods are

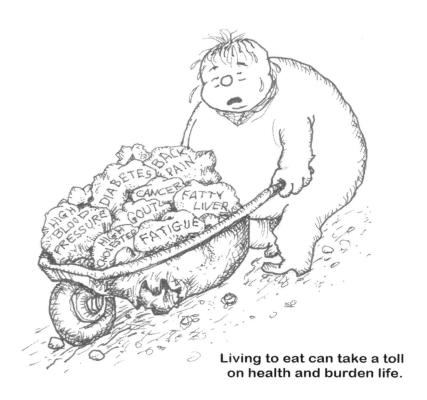

Living to eat can take a toll on health and burden life.

usually dense in fat and protein calories. If you want to eat until you are full, then your meal should contain a certain percentage of low calorie fruits and vegetables. These foods will fill you up without overloading your body with extra calories.

Overeating or being too full is not healthy. Overeating can cause nausea, vomiting, stomach discomfort, pain, cramps and serious illnesses, such as acid reflex, acute or chronic gastritis and acute pancreatitis. An ancient Chinese saying claims that it will take the span of ten meals to recover from one overly full belly. Some chronic digestive disorders, like acid reflex or gastritis, may be caused by the bad habit of overeating. If you have these digestive disorders, then you should eat five or six small meals every day, instead of three larger meals.

Not eating enough can also cause health problems. For example, if you do not get enough food or nutrition, you can develop a nutritional deficiency. Being hungry often can also cause digestive disorders, such as IBS, food intolerance, gastritis, colitis and can lead to anorexia. When you are hungry too often, digestive enzymes are not stimulated. Eating stimulates enzymes and maintains the ability of your digestive tract to function properly. Being hungry can lower the digestive system's immune ability, making it easier to develop food intolerance and constipation. It is important to eat regularly. If you are worried that you will gain weight, then eat low calorie foods.

Eating regularly is necessary in order to properly stimulate the digestive tract. Skipping meals or not eating regularly can cause digestive disorders. The hardest thing for your stomach to handle is to skip one meal when you are hungry and then eat a big meal later. This can cause serious digestive disorders and I have found it to be the most common cause of acid reflex and IBS for my patients. The common suggestion is to eat three meals a day. However, eating five or six smaller meals throughout the day is better for your digestion than eating three big meals, especially for people who already have a digestive disorder.

Every meal –breakfast, lunch and dinner should contain different amounts and types of food. If you are able to eat five or six smaller meals each day, then simply break your portions for each meal in half and eat them over two meals instead of one.

Breakfast should be a large meal (the largest meal of the day by volume) containing easy to digest starches, such as rice or oatmeal, fruit, and a large amount of fluids. In the morning you are dehydrated after sleep, so you need plenty of water, and some easy to digest glucose rich, simple starchy foods. These glucose rich foods will provide you with 1818energy for the day. Eating these foods is a better way to get energized than by drinking coffee or other caffeinated beverages.

Lunch should be smaller portioned than breakfast, but should contain more calorie dense food. This can be achieved by eating high calorie foods, such as meat or dairy. Lunch should be smaller portioned, because eating too much may cause drowsiness in the afternoon.

Dinner should be the smallest meal of the day, especially if you eat less than three hours before going to bed. If you eat earlier, you can eat a larger meal. For example, if you eat a large meal at five o'clock and you go to bed at ten o'clock, your body has enough time to digest the food. But, if you eat a small meal at five o'clock, you might be hungry by the time you are ready to go to bed, and it is not good to go to bed hungry. Again, you may choose to eat a small meal in the early evening and then eat a small meal no later than three hours before going to bed. You should not feel too full after dinner. If you go to bed full, your stomach will be stretched too long (because your ability to process food slows down during sleep) and can cause discomfort that may affect the quality of your sleep. This can lead to digestive disorders.

Big Question 3: How Can I Lower My Appetite?

This is another very frequent question my patients ask me. They often tell me that they always feel hungry, especially when they are trying to lose weight by eating less. My personal answer to this question is that consuming more liquids and water dense foods will help cut down your appetite. The less you eat, the less appetite you will have. The two main reasons for this is that feeling full actually physically stimulates your digestive system, intensifying the sensation of wanting to eat more and the presence of food in your digestive system signals the production of enzymes that increases your appetite as well. The act of chewing also prompts the stimulation of digestive enzymes and physically stimulates your digestive tract.

If you want to lose weight, you can drink more liquid food to cut down your appetite. My advice is to add low sodium soups and water rich foods, such as oatmeal, rice, etc. to your diet as a way to start reducing your appetite. If you have a poor digestive system already, or you feel ill, then you should chew more food and try to avoid drinking your food. Liquid foods that don't require chewing, such as soups, can lower your appetite and may further disrupt existing digestive ailments. Drinking food will not stimulate your digestive system too much and because of this, drinking foods long-term can cause indigestion, IBS and long-term loss of appetite. If you fail to eat and chew foods over a long period of time, your digestion will not function as well and you will feel discomfort, gas and bloating.

A person's appetite level can be affected by their diet. The motion of chewing food will stimulate your digestive system. The process of digestion begins in your mouth with your saliva. Chewing can increase your appetite. If you want to increase your appetite, then chew slowly and eat more dry foods. From my experience there are generally four levels of appetite that most people fit into to as follows.

1. *Overactive appetite* –people with overactive appetite eat until they are physically full but still feel hungry. These people may have hormone disorders (for example, hyperthyroidism), uncontrolled diabetes or may be taking steroids. People with overactive appetite may snack a lot. The more you snack, especially dry food, such as crackers and chips, the hungrier you become because chewing stimulates your digestive system.

2. *Normal appetite* –people who feel hungry, eat and then feel satisfied have a normal appetite.

3. *Changing appetite* –people with an appetite level that changes will feel very hungry some days and will have little or no appetite on other days. This is a well-known symptom of IBS. People who suffer from IBS often feel hungry, but after eating, they feel discomfort in their digestive system, such as bloating, cramps, gas or even diarrhea. Sometimes people with this kind of appetite will be afraid to eat because they know eating can cause them pain and discomfort.

4. *Little to no appetite* –people who do not want to eat or are afraid to eat have no appetite. (This may happen occasionally when someone is sick for some reason, such as the flu.) Some people can look at or smell food and feel nauseous. Sometimes just the thought of eating creates fear and discomfort for some people. When this is a chronic condition it is known as anorexia. Anorexia starts as a disease associated with emotional disorders; however, lack of eating becomes a physical disease as well when anorexia causes your digestive system to stop working. If the condition is left untreated, a person suffering from anorexia may not be able to physically digest food. Anorexia is a serious, potentially life-threatening disease that requires immediate medical care.

Big Question 4: What Types of Food Should I Eat?

Whenever one of my patients asks me how much they should eat, they also ask me what type of foods they should eat. Individual foods cannot meet all of your body's nutritional needs. We have to eat a wide variety of foods to meet our nutritional needs. But, as I explained earlier, this does not mean the larger variety of food, the better. Remember that allergies and food intolerances are very common, so regardless of how healthy a food is, if you are unable to tolerate a certain food, it is important to avoid eating it. The healthiest food is not always healthy for everyone. Here is some nutritional information about common foods.

Whole Grains

Whole grain foods contain mostly starches; including resistant starch.[1] Whole grains contain a small percent of protein, fiber, vitamins and minerals. Whole grain foods are not as tasty as dairy, meat or other high calorie foods. Eating whole grain foods is less problematic for your cholesterol levels precisely because they are not high in calories, like animal fat and highly concentrated sugary foods. This does not mean that if you only eat whole grain foods you will not get high cholesterol, diabetes or high blood pressure; if you eat too many calories of any food, you will run into health issues. For example, bread can be made from whole grain, but bread is still high in calories. If you eat too much bread you can develop metabolic syndrome.

Whole grains are rich in fiber. Fiber is necessary for the stimulation of your digestive system. Eating enough fiber maintains the digestive system's motion (peristalsis) and helps clean out the digestive system, especially the colon. Fiber cannot be broken down or digested, but it can stimulate the digestive system and allow enough pressure build up in the colon to cause regular bowel movements. Not eating enough fiber can lead to constipation, which can cause colon cancer and colitis. Whole grain foods can also be environmentally friendly, unlike dairy and meat, the production of which causes a lot of pollution.[2] If you eat a variety of whole grains and vegetables and get enough sunshine, you can get almost all of the nutrition your body requires with the exception of some essential minerals such as salt. This is why veganism can be a healthy lifestyle choice. In Asia and most developing countries, rice and wheat are the main foods. Whole grains are some of the healthiest energy sources. Adding them to your diet can help you maintain good health.

Most Americans do not consider whole grains to be healthy foods because they are high in calories and carbohydrates. Although bread can be unhealthy, it is unhealthy for reasons other than its calorie count. In actuality, most bread is cooked to the point where it is burnt. If bread is browned, then it is burnt. Burnt grains contain carcinogens that may cause cancer.[3] When cooked until brown, bread becomes dry, which can over stimulate the appetite because of the extra chewing required. Also, if you add unhealthy condiments to bread, such as salt, sugar, dairy or margarine, the bread becomes unhealthy. Bread is a good source of necessary glucose. However, some people have celiac disease, an allergy to wheat products. For these people, even a small amount of gluten can create severe health consequences. This is another example of why it is impossible to recommend that certain foods are the best foods or healthy for everyone.

Rice

Rice should be considered part of a healthy diet. Rice is mainly water and carbohydrates that are turned into glucose in the body. Glucose is the body's fuel, we need glucose to operate in daily life; rice supplies plenty of glucose. Also, because cooked rice is mainly water, it is not that high in calories. Rice alone is boring, so it is unlikely that you will eat too much rice. It does not provide all of the nutrition we need, but it does provide a necessary amount of resistant starch. As is well known, the main cause of diabetes is the overconsumption of high calorie foods, such as meat and refined sugar. So, even if you are diabetic, a normal servicing of rice shouldn't cause concern for your glucose intake. Additionally, only a very small amount of people are allergic or intolerant to rice. Because rice is boiled or steamed, and not usually eaten if burnt, it is healthier for your diet than bread.

White rice contains about thirteen percent protein (about four grams per serving). Brown rice contains slightly more protein per serving at about seventeen per serving.[4] Rice is a good source of necessary amino acids. Rice is the main food in the world, especially in developing countries. Personally, I eat white rice almost every day and with nearly every meal.

Other Grains and Soy

Other whole grain foods such as beans and millet contain much more protein than rice and wheat. There is such a large variety of grain foods available that you should find it easy to try different whole grains. Once you find ones that you enjoy and can tolerate, it will be easy for you to add them to your diet. If you require a high protein diet, soy beans provide a good source of protein. One serving of soybeans can provide more than fifty percent of the daily recommended value of protein for an average adult. Soybeans contain the highest percentage of protein of all crop foods.[5] Protein from soy may be a better choice than meat for you if you have high cholesterol, blood pressure or diabetes.

Keep in mind, however, that soy is still a calorie rich grain. Soy is one of the most common food allergies and intolerance triggers in children.[6] Soy is difficult to be break down and digest and, therefore, can cause gas, bloating and indigestion. If eaten raw or not fully cooked, soybeans can be toxic because they contain phylates, which act as an anti-nutrient and block the body's absorption of minerals from the gastrointestinal tract. This chemical can also cause the pancreas to swell. It is important to only eat soy and soybeans that have been properly cooked. There are many sources of information that provide studies on soy in the diet. You may find that studies performed in Asia and America has strikingly different results. You may research this topic further if you are concerned about the possible effects of soy in your diet. However, I advise that you use discernment when choosing which sources of information to trust. If possible, look for broad-based studies sponsored by national not-for-profit health organizations rather than by for-profit organizations.

Meat

Meat (animal flesh consumed for food) contains fat, protein and a small amount of vitamins and minerals. Because meat is high in calories, it takes longer to become hungry after eating it; so people feel more satisfied after eating meat rich meals. A bellyful of meat can last you up to eight hours, whereas a bellyful of rice and vegetables can for about four or five hours. Many people say that they do not feel satisfied after eating Chinese food because it mainly rice and vegetables and contains less meat. People who burn a lot of calories by working hard physically, exercising often or playing extreme competitive sports can eat plenty of meat and not worry about their caloric intake. A small amount of meat can be used to flavor a large amount of stir-fried vegetables. When you eat vegetables with meat your digestion is better able to absorb the nutrition of the vegetables. For example, vitamin A and E is only absorbed when combined with some type of fat. If you are underweight, you should eat more meat to gain weight.

Meat is mostly fat and protein and is high in calories. People think meat is merely high in protein, but the truth is that the majority of meat contains a large percentage of the recommended daily intake of fat as well. It is easy to eat too much meat because of its density and flavor. If you eat only meat you may gain weight or develop other health problems. Most people today work at a desk, even farmers spend the majority of their time sitting; these days very few jobs require intense physical work. But, people eat as if they do a lot of physical activity during the day. Only if you have an active job (or exercise for long periods of time) can you burn the necessary amount of calories required to burn off the excess energy created by having too much meat in your diet. The idea of meat and potatoes as a meal became traditional for the hard laboring man –not today's office worker.

Eating too much meat (consuming too many calories) is the main cause of metabolic syndrome and being overweight. When I was growing up in China, very few families, especially in the countryside, could afford to eat meat; the average person could only have one meal with meat once per month. At that time, there was a very low rate of diabetes and high blood pressure in China. In fact, it was almost never heard of. But, today, because the economy has improved, people can afford to eat meat every day. This has caused the obesity, diabetes and high blood pressure rates in China to skyrocket.[7] Our mentality towards meat may be stuck in the past; we do not need to eat a lot of meat to sustain ourselves. You need to count calories and eat the amount of meat calories that you need to meet your health requirements –not eat how much you want.

Unfortunately, it is difficult to be this self-disciplined. Most people fail to achieve this level of self-discipline. A lot of people claim that a surplus intake of sugar causes diabetes, but the reality is that meat, because of its high caloric count, causes far more cases of diabetes than sugar does. I have observed this reality for the last fifteen years in my practice. As another example, as I said earlier, diabetes was a rare disease when I was growing up in China. At that time people ate a lot of corn, cornbread and other breads (foods high in glucose), but because they rarely ate any meat, the diabetes rate stayed low. A diabetic's glucose level will not rise as quickly from eating meat as it will from drinking a glass of apple juice. But, in the long-run, eating a lot of meat over time will cause your glucose to steadily rise, remain high and worsen your diabetes. This is because your body turns unused calories into glucose. If you consume more calories than you need, even the calories are consumed from protein; your body will have to process more glucose than it needs possibly leading to metabolic syndrome and diabetes. If you are overweight or have metabolic syndrome, you should limit your intake of meat. It is not meat itself that causes diabetes or other health issues, but rather the amount that is eaten. Remember, food is not supposed to be used for entertainment. Food is nourishment and medicine. Hippocrates, the father of western medicine said, "Let food by thy medicine and medicine be thy food." That advice is still valid today.

Meat increases bad cholesterol. Animal fat contains bad cholesterol (LDL). The body can turn even the leanest meat, if eaten in quantities too large for your body and health needs, into bad cholesterol. People forget that we, ourselves, are animals. If you already have high cholesterol, be extra cautious with your meat intake.

The way meat is generally cooked in America is unhealthy. The most common ways to cook meat in America are by grilling, frying and smoking. Browning and blackening meat is actually burning meat, which creates carcinogens.[8] Additionally, the gas used to cook (whether for indoor grills or stoves or for outdoor grills), although it adds flavor, creates a lot of toxins that can cause cancer and other health problems.[9] Boiling meat (like boiling meat in beef stew) and moist-baking at lower temperatures are much better ways to cook meat.

Sausage, hot dogs, jerky, canned meat, bacon and lunch or deli meats are highly processed. When these forms of meat are produced, the majority of manufacturers put a high amount of preservatives and additives in them. (Not to mention that the main ingredients actually used to make most processed meats are the leftovers from the slaughterhouse floor. Many manufacturers essentially add bleach to these meats in order to reduce the amount of bacteria in them.[10]) Additionally, because of how these meats are processed, they contain more nitrates and most companies add nitrates in order to give their products a longer shelf life. If you cut one piece of a sausage or hotdog and leave it at room temperature (not in the refrigerator) it will not rot. We need to use our common sense here. If meat does not rot when left outside, this means that germs, which are living organisms, cannot eat this food. This is a sign that we should not eat this food either. If we eat too much processed meat, who knows what it will do to our bodies. Remember, the body is a living system composed of varying forms of good and bad bacteria and germs. You have probably heard of fast food hamburgers that don't rot even after being left at room temperature for months. Consider, for the sake of your health –if microorganisms (germs) will not eat a food, then we probably shouldn't either.

Meat is greasy and tasty. It is a natural instinct to want to eat greasy, heavy foods. It has been speculated that our ancestors never knew when or where their next meal would come from, so they would eat foods that would sustain them for long periods of time, that is, the greasiest, highest energy foods that they could find. Now, eating meat is used as a form of entertainment. When people go out to restaurants they almost always order meat. Meat is a satisfying, and sometimes, addictive food that gives us energy. If you are used to eating meat often, it will be hard to incorporate rice and vegetables into your diet.

Improper feed supplied to livestock such as hormones, antibiotics, pesticides, medications, etc. can affect the quality of the food you eat. Clenbuterol (an anabolic steroid) has been known to be fed to animals in order to produce leaner meat cuts. There are known cases of this additive causing severe illness (food poisoning) in people who have eaten meat from animals who were fed this medication.[11]

Medications can give animals side effects like heart problems, just as they can for us. If an animal has been given too much medication, a person can get food poisoning from eating the meat of that animal.[12] When you eat meat that was fed growth hormones, steroids, antibiotics, anti-worm drugs, antiparasitics, pesticide or herbicide-laced feed, etc., you are essentially feeding yourself those additives as well. Antibiotics are commonly given to livestock for preventative measures because conditions are so polluted and unhealthy that the animals need antibiotics just to stay alive. Dosing animals with antibiotics is cheaper than providing sanitary living conditions for these "products."[13] The addition of growth hormones has been linked to girls starting to menstruate much earlier than in the past. Girls as young as nine have been forced into early puberty because of the additives that are in the food they are fed.[14]

Some people have trouble digesting meat, so use extra caution and listen to your body. It should be easy to figure out if you are intolerant to a certain type of meat.

After an animal has been butchered, it is common for the meat to be aged. Aging meat in order to make it more tender and flavorful is achieved by hanging meat for about one to three weeks. Sometimes, individual cuts of meat are packaged and then aged for several weeks. Enzymes break down muscle tissue during the aging process –aging is the intentional rotting of meat. During the aging process nitrite and nitrate toxins build up in the meat; these toxins can create severe health problems for children and are known to increase cancer risk in adults.[15] Aging meat makes meat tender, tasty and unhealthy.

In order to keep meat fresh and appealing, manufacturers and producers add preservatives, food coloring, bacteria, etc. to meat. Radiation may also be used as a way to preserve and kill bad bacteria in meat.[16] It may be argued that some methods make the meat supply initially safer because E.coli and other potentially deadly organisms are killed by some of these processes.[17]

Modern food production is indeed a marvel. Starvation in the modern world has been virtually eradicated. Our food supply is consistent and offers year-round variety of all types of foods. We no longer have to depend on our own crop production in order to eat and we don't have to worry about crop failures as much. However, we are talking about long-term health. Short-term gains for a safer food supply are achieved at the risk or sacrifice of our long-term health caused by repeated, internal exposure to nitrites, radiation, antibiotics, chemicals, etc.

When I was a child, only fresh meat was eaten. If we had a special occasion to eat meat, the livestock was often slaughtered, prepared and eaten within a few hours. Even today in China and other developing countries it is still common to see livestock on display at shops and restaurants. A lack of refrigeration in these areas has required that meat and fish be kept alive until purchased for a meal. An unintentional side benefit of this practice is that this meat is served very fresh and does not have time to spoil. Unfortunately, having a reliable and modern food supply does have some disadvantages for our health. We have to ship meat, wrap it in plastics, display in stores, freeze it, etc. By the time a person eats the meat, six months to a year or more may have passed since the meat was initially prepared for the food supply. Fresh meat is the best choice for your health, but most people today could not tolerate to eat meat if they had to view the butchering process.

After we research the facts for ourselves, we should be able to determine that meat should not be blindly considered as a healthy foundation of our diet. We can make informed choices as to which types of meat we eat and chose fresh meats that contain less or no additives and that have been raised responsibly.

Vegetables

Vegetables are rich in healthy fiber, water, minerals, vitamins, antioxidants and contain small amounts of protein and starch.[18] Fiber is not broken down by our digestive system and does not provide much nutrition. But, fiber is important for our diet because it stimulates our digestive tracts and maintains normal intestinal motion by creating pressure in the colon that encourages regular bowel movements, which prevents constipation and accumulation of toxins in the body. Although fiber cannot be broken down, it can still fill us up and make us feel full, which is important for our digestive health. Vegetables can make us feel full, thereby complementing our modern life in which there is little physical work required of us. Fiber rich vegetables can prevent us from becoming overweight and developing health problems, such as metabolic syndrome.

Half of the majority of your meals should be made up of vegetables in order to avoid consuming too many calories. Vegetables are the richest, healthiest mineral source of food available and are also rich in various vitamins, such as A, C and E and antioxidants that help slow the aging process. Vegetables are an important part of a healthy diet. Vegetables contain few calories, but because they contain fiber, can fill us up and promote normal digestive motion. Eating a diet high in fiber is a healthy choice for persons who have physically inactive careers or lifestyles.

Like any food, all vegetables are not good for everyone. Different people will be able to tolerate different vegetables. Because vegetables do not contain many calories, it is not good for people who are underweight or have poor appetites to eat mainly vegetables. Some people experience discomfort from eating high fiber foods, and most people have some sort of intolerance to one or more vegetable (the intolerance rate for vegetables is high). Intolerance to vegetables and fiber can cause bloating, gas, indigestion, cramps and diarrhea. People that have stomach problems, such as IBS or a weak digestive system, should be extra cautious about eating vegetables. For example, onions, garlic and leeks have the highest intolerance rates for the average person. These foods can cause gas, heartburn, bloating and diarrhea. Spicy vegetables, such as hot peppers, can also irritate your digestive system. Certain vegetables can cause some people to experience excessive bloating and gas. Pay attention to which vegetables cause you discomfort and stay away from them. Some people in the Western world are not used to eating a large amount of vegetables, so eating a lot of veggies at one meal can cause digestive discomfort. It is common for raw vegetables to create more intolerances than cooked vegetables. Cooking vegetables by steaming or lightly frying and properly flavoring them with animal fat or oil can make them easier to digest and allow their nutrients to be better absorbed by our bodies.

Cooking fresh vegetables is best. The longer vegetables are stored the more nitrates they accumulate. During the natural rotting process, mold and other organisms grow on vegetables creating nitrates. The rotting process is accelerated by cooking or marinating these foods. Many people will cook large meals and store leftovers to eat throughout the week, but after only two days, leftovers may already contain too many nitrates to be considered safe to eat. It is best to cook and eat vegetables immediately and not keep them for the next day's meal.

Many people, especially children, feel that vegetables are not tasty, especially raw vegetables. Most people do not go to restaurants and order vegetables because they are not very flavorful. In order to make vegetables tasty we can flavor them with animal meat and spices. Asia's main cooking technique, stir-frying, is an excellent way to make vegetables tasty. You can look up recipes online or pick up a cookbook on Asian cooking to learn how to make vegetables tasty.
Grilling, marinating and cooking vegetables for too long can cause them to not only lose their nutritional value, but can make them toxic if eaten.

People need to be careful when growing vegetables. When growing a large amount of one type of food (monoculture), insects and pests can become a problem, so a lot of farmers use herbicides and pesticides. Using chemical fertilizers can increase the nitrate level in vegetables. Organic foods and garden-raised vegetables do not contain these toxic chemicals, so they are much better for your health.

Juicing vegetables has become a popular health habit in America. Adequate nutrition is vital, but like anything, too much nutrition is bad for your health. It is possible for vegetable juices to contain too many vitamins and minerals. It may take four or five pounds of cabbage to make one glass of cabbage juice. Drinking juice causes you to ingest an increased amount of acid and minerals, which can cause bloating, gas and diarrhea; most people have diarrhea after drinking too much vegetable juice. If you can tolerate the juice without getting diarrhea, it is likely that you will develop a kidney stone.

The fact is that vegetable juice may simply contain too much nutrition and oxalic acid[19] for your body to process at one time. Chewing stimulates enzymes, so drinking vegetable juice will not stimulate your digestive system. Also, it is common for raw vegetables to have bacteria present on their skins. Cooking vegetables kills the majority of the bad bacteria that juicing cannot. Because the liquid content in vegetable juice is so high, your stomach acid is less effective at killing bacteria; this may increase your chance of becoming ill from eating uncooked vegetables. There is a small percentage of the population that is allergic to vegetables. Some people will feel itchiness, swelling or mouth ulcers when they eat certain vegetables, but severe allergies to vegetables are rare.

Fruits

Fruits contain mostly water, some fiber, minerals and vitamins, a small amount of protein and a lot of natural sugars. Most fruits are low calorie foods. But some fruits, such as figs, coconuts and bananas should be viewed as higher calorie foods.

Fruits contain a lot of natural sugars. These sugars create pleasant fragrances and delicious tastes, but can also make fruit addictive for some people. Fruit does not contain a large amount of nutrition, so eating fruit will not provide you with the proper nutrition that you need. This is especially true for children. Young people, underweight people, persons with illnesses and the elderly should not eat too much fruit in order to ensure they are meeting all of their nutritional needs by eating a variety of foods. In general, because fruits contain mostly water, eating a bellyful of fruit will not cause you too many problems, unless you have diabetes because fruit sugars can cause your glucose level to rise.

Most fruits contain acid. Fruit acids are the main cause of tooth cavities. Fruit lovers will most likely develop cavities from eating sour fruit. After eating fruit, it is good to rinse your mouth with a simple mixture of baking soda and water as a way to prevent cavities. The acid and sweetness in fruit, especially in fruit juice, can also cause acid reflux. Some acid can be poisonous. For example, unripen apricots or plums can be poisonous and many people are intolerant to the high level of acid present in unripe fruits. Even bugs tend not to eat these highly acidic fruits because they are so sour and toxic. Some people do not eat fruit because it is too tart, but fruit is sour because it is not yet ripe. It is more pleasant to eat ripened fruit. Farmers have to pick fruit early and factor in shipping time so that fruit is not visibly rotting by the time it arrives at the market. But, if fruit is full of acid, to the point where bacteria will not eat it, then it will be harsh on your digestive system. Your digestive system contains both good and bad bacteria. Good bacterium is crucial for your digestive system to be able to function properly. If the bacteria in your digestive tract are not able to break down the acid in the fruit you eat, then you will experience digestive discomfort and possibly other digestive problems.

Fruit must be eaten fresh. Like vegetables, the longer you store fruit, the more nitrates will be produced. After a certain point, fruit will be more poisonous than beneficial. In fact, rotted fruit can cause digestive disorders and may be carcinogenic.[20] Unfortunately, about fifty percent of the fruit found in the stores is rotted. When one part of the apple is rotted, you should assume that the rest of the apple is already contaminated by nitrates or is on the verge of rotting. So, it is better to not eat partially rotted fruit. The best place to store fruit is in the refrigerator; this will delay the rotting process. Most people assume that if a fruit is sweet then it is not rotted; but rotted apples and bananas are much sweeter than ripened apples and bananas.

Some fruits are natural laxatives such as berries, cherries and plums. Eating too much of these fruits can cause bloating and diarrhea. If you already have digestive issues, eat these fruits in moderation.

Fruit is a common culprit of food allergies and intolerances. Citrus fruits, such as pineapple, oranges and lemons commonly cause mouth ulcers and anal rashes in people who are sensitive or allergic to them. Allergy reactions or intolerances to strawberries and bananas are also common. You may notice that you develop symptoms after eating certain types of fruits, if this is the case, avoid eating these fruits and notice if your symptoms go and stay away.

Eating fruit is better than drinking fruit juice. The fiber in fruit is good for your digestive tract, but fruit juice may contain too much sugar. Fruit contains essential vitamins and minerals. For example, we only need two to three oranges a day to get the vitamin C required for one day, but when juicing oranges, it may take a dozen oranges to make one glass of juice. Since fruit contains so much sugar, diabetics should avoid drinking fruit juice so that their glucose levels don't rise too quickly. Fruit skin contains the most nutrition and minerals, but it is hard to find fruit that has not been sprayed with pesticides. Apples and peaches are favored by pests, so farmers have to spray a lot of toxic chemicals on them to keep the bugs away; these sprays are not good for us either. Pesticides, fungicides and herbicides are not easy to wash off and often fruits rot from the inside out because there are so many chemicals preserving the surface of the fruit. If you do not eat organic fruit it is better to peel the skin off. (Some pesticides are applied systemically, that is, the tree is treated at the root and the chemicals travel throughout the tree and into the fruit. So, when possible, choose organic fruits.) Fruit is healthy, but this doesn't mean that you should eat a lot of it. Fruit juice bought in stores is not good for you because of its high sugar content. Whenever possible, dilute pure fruit juices with water; this will reduce the sugar and calorie content of your serving. Some store-bought juices contain preservatives, additives and food coloring; these juices should not be considered healthy additions to your diet.

Some people eat fruit seeds, because they think they contain more nutrition. However, some seeds can be toxic. For example, apricot seeds and cherry seeds contain cyanide compounds. If an adult swallows a couple seeds there is no cause for concern, but children and pets can be poisoned by these toxic compounds. If you have diverticulitis you should not eat fruits with tiny seeds, such as pomegranate seeds or seeded grapes. Diverticulitis is caused by the formation of pouches on the outside of the large intestine. Diverticulitis is an extremely painful condition. These pockets can easily become inflamed if a seed is trapped in one of them.

Dried fruits contain the same amount of nutrition as fresh fruit, but are actually higher in calories per serving. It is easy to eat too much dried fruit, such as raisins. If you are overweight you should pay attention to how many dried fruit calories you consume. Also, be aware that some dried fruits contain high amounts of preservatives.

Most fruits should be eaten fresh and should not be cooked. Types of cooked fruit include jams, jellies, canned fruit, fruit added to baked goods, etc. Fresh fruits are rich in antioxidants. Because of the reasons I have just explained, you can understand why I do not consider fruit to be part of a healthy diet. If you do eat fruit it is important to do so moderately. Eat fresh, high quality organic produce whenever possible.

Fish and Seafood

Seafood includes ocean fish, freshwater fish and shellfish. Fish are rich in protein, healthy fats, minerals and vitamins and are considered an important part of a healthy diet. Fish contains heart healthy unsaturated fatty acids including omega 3. Fish, especially deep ocean seafood, such as salmon and halibut, can raise your HDL level, the good cholesterol that protects your arteries from LDL (bad cholesterol) damage and slows down the process of arteriosclerosis. This is why cultures that traditionally consume a lot of fish, such as the Japanese, tend to have higher life expectancies. Fish is easy to digest and is easily absorbed by the body, causing less trouble for the digestive system than meat, which is why seafood is good for older people and those who have digestive disorders, such as IBS. Fish contains more minerals and vitamins, such as vitamins A, E and D and calcium than any meat. Even though fish has many health benefits, it can cause health problems as well. There are important factors to consider when adding fish to your diet.

First of all, fish is a calorie rich food, so overconsumption of fish can easily lead to being over nourished which can cause weight gain, diabetes and high cholesterol problems. Compared to animal fat and meat, seafood can be part a healthy diet, but extra seafood calories are just as lethal to our health; extra glucose can easily be turned into bad cholesterol. For example, one of my diabetic patients went on an ocean cruise and ate a lot of seafood for two weeks. She experienced a rise in her glucose level and told me that she couldn't understand why her glucose level rose when she hadn't had many carbohydrates. I explained to her that an increase in her caloric intake, even though it was from a protein source, caused her glucose level to rise. Another patient of mine had a cholesterol problem and learned that seafood could increase his good cholesterol. He started to consume a lot of fish and his good cholesterol did rise slightly, but his bad cholesterol rose as well. His total cholesterol count increased simply because he was consuming more calories than his body needed.

Fish must be fresh. Seafood spoils easily, especially in warmer temperatures. When fish spoils, a higher concentration of histamine and nitrates develop in it. It is important to store fish properly. Freezing fish is usually the best way to preserve it. You can use your sense of smell to determine the freshness of fish. The smellier the fish, the less fresh it is. Some people cannot tolerate the smell of fish, but if fish is fresh, then the smell will not be strong. Salted, marinated and dried fish smell the worst and it is no surprise that these forms of fish are the most concentrated with nitrates. Most people buy "fresh" fish from the supermarket, but it is most likely that this fish is not fresh, especially in locations that are inland and offshore. First, fish has to be caught, butchered, shipped to the store, placed on display for sale and then, after being bought, is usually stored in the refrigerator for a few days before being cooked. The freshest seafood you can get from the store is fish that has arrived at the store frozen.

Cooked seafood is best. Seafood is often contaminated with viruses, bacteria and parasites. Deep ocean fish can be eaten raw, but only with caution. It is much more likely to get food poisoning from raw fish than from cooked fish. It is easier to get food-borne illness from fish that hasn't been cooked including illnesses caused by improper preparation and handling like hepatitis A.

Some fish live in water that is polluted with heavy metals, pesticides, fertilizer and medication; eating this fish causes you to ingest these toxins. For example, if you go fishing in an area surrounded by a lot of traffic, then the fish you catch will most likely contain more heavy metals (lead or mercury); fish caught from a secluded lake will most likely be much healthier. Shellfish are bottom feeders. They will eat practically anything on the ocean floor; they are like filters for the ocean floor. So, shellfish that come from ocean shores or bays that are in close proximity to big cities may be contaminated by pollution. You need to be extra cautious when you buy or catch shellfish. If you eat a clam that has sand in it, the sand can bother your teeth and can cause or increase your chances of having appendicitis. It is important to buy fish from local fishermen who know what is in season. For example, in Alaska, there is a certain clam that can be very toxic depending on the season. Talk to local fishermen to learn about what is edible and in season in your area.

A high percentage of people have allergic reactions to seafood, especially shellfish. It is estimated that about 2.3% of the U.S. population is allergic to shellfish[21] and 6.5 million people are allergic to seafood, which is more than double the amount of people dealing with nut allergies.[22] The most common symptoms of seafood allergies are skin rashes and hives. Histamine in canned or old seafood can cause adverse reactions that are similar to allergic reactions.

Nuts

Nuts are rich in fatty acids, protein and contain starch, minerals and vitamins, especially vitamin B. Nuts are considered a healthy source of protein for most people. In ancient China people recognized that the walnut is shaped like the brain, so they believed that eating one to two walnuts a day was good for the brain. We now know that nuts have lecithin, a special fat and nutrition source that our brains need. Like anything else, nuts need to be eaten moderately and prepared correctly.

Nuts are high in calories and fat. Eating too many nuts can cause health problems. So, it is important to count calories when eating nuts, and not just treat them as a guilt-free snack. It is best to only eat a few nuts at a time.

Nuts are difficult to digest, break down and absorb. Many people are intolerant to nuts. Intolerance or eating too many nuts can cause nausea, gas and bloating. Tree nuts and peanuts both have high allergy rates. About three million Americans are allergic to peanuts[23] and almost two million Americans are allergic to tree nuts.[24] The most common allergy reaction to nuts is a burning feeling in the tongue, itchy tonsils and a swollen throat which can threaten the air supply; serious reactions to nuts include anaphylactic shock, diarrhea and vomiting. People who are allergic to nuts should be extra cautious and pay attention to all of the ingredients listed in the food they eat.

Nuts can be easily contaminated and rotted. Like other foods, when rotted or molded, nuts contain more nitrates and toxins that can cause cancer and affect the digestive system. The nuts most susceptible to rotting are sunflower seeds and peanuts. Peanuts are grown in warm, moist climates; if not harvested in time, handled, processed or stored properly they can easily rot. It is best to buy raw peanuts, because it is much easier to tell whether or not they have spoiled just by visually inspecting them for mold and decay. You can also tell whether or not a nut has spoiled by the taste because it will taste unpleasant or different than you would expect that particular type of nut to taste. Peanuts are often turned into peanut butter. Because of the processing, it is close to impossible to tell whether or not peanut butter has spoiled. It is best to make your own peanut butter or sunflower seed butter. Many people enjoy roasted nuts, but high temperatures can burn nuts. Burnt nuts contain more carcinogens (most whole grain health bars tend to contain rotted or overcooked nuts). The healthiest way to eat nuts is to buy and eat them raw or prepare them yourself.

Young children should not eat nuts. Children are not as experienced with chewing, so if they are laughing, crying or are very excited, a part of the nut can be lodged into the back of their throat in the windpipe and cause serious problems. This is a common cause of children's visits to the emergency room. It is best to give older children nut butter as opposed to hard nuts. The most common recommendation is to never give a child under five years of age nuts (or other small food pieces) that may be choking hazards.[25, 26] Some people choose not to give children under five years of age nuts as a way to prevent or reduce their risk of developing a nut allergy. It is commonly acknowledged that children under three years of age should not be given peanut butter or other peanut products.[27]

Dairy Products

In some countries and cultures, such as America, dairy products have become a key part of what is considered to be a healthy diet. Dairy products contain nearly all the nutrition the body needs. Dairy is easily digested and absorbed and is good for infants and young children, older people and people who have digestive issues and nutritional deficiencies. Dairy includes milk, cheese, yogurt and cream.

Dairy products, such as cheese, are incredibly rich in calories. It is important for adults to be deliberate about moderating their serving sizes of dairy products because dairy foods are easily digested; therefore, eating too much dairy may lead to overconsumption and overnutrition (weight gain).

Even though dairy is easily digested, it is also the number one food group that causes food intolerance and allergies in adults. It has been estimated that between thirty and fifty million American adults are either intolerant or allergic to dairy.[28] The most common digestive condition related to dairy is known as lactose intolerance. Lactose intolerance can cause bloating, gas, diarrhea, nasal allergies, asthma and autoimmune disorders. Dairy protein molecules can be easily absorbed through the intestine into the blood stream. For those who are intolerant or allergic, the protein can trigger the body to mistakenly identify the protein as a foreign substance, and in response develop antibodies to attack the dairy protein. If you have an autoimmune disease, you should have an allergy test to make sure you are not allergic to dairy.

Eating dairy that has been cooked for too long (crunchy and browned cheese most commonly found on pizza) is toxic and not good for your health. Processed dairy can be problematic as well. For example, cheese contains histamine and nitrates which can cause hives, headaches and flare-up existing skin conditions, such as psoriasis. When milk is processed, chemicals and additives are usually added to the milk to prolong its shelf life and improve its taste. These added substances can cause health problems. For example, the 2008 Chinese milk scandal was caused by the additive melamine. The contamination compromised the well-being of millions of children, resulted in the death of at least four babies, over fifty three thousand ill children and about six thousand cases of children hospitalized for kidney disease.[29]

As with all food, organic dairy products are better. The majority of non-organic dairy farmers give their cows antibiotics in order to prevent infections.[30] The antibiotics inevitably will be secreted into the dairy products that are produced and may cause distress to your digestive system.

Eggs

Eggs, mainly chicken eggs, are a very popular part of the American diet (in other countries people also eat duck eggs and quail eggs). Eggs, like dairy, have more vitamins and minerals than chicken meat. Eggs are one of the few foods that contain nearly all of the nutrition our bodies need. Because of this, eggs are good for children, the elderly, people who have digestive problems, people with poor appetites and people who are suffering from illnesses.

Eggs are high in calories because they contain a lot of fat and protein. Generally speaking, America is facing an overnutrition problem, not a nutritional deficiency problem. So, it is probably best for people who are trying to manage their caloric intake to use eggs as part of their diet, but not as a main part of their diet. Yolks are especially calorie and cholesterol dense. Eating one or two eggs everyday as part of a healthy, balanced diet should be fine for most people.

Egg nutrition varies depending on the chicken feed and living conditions of the chickens. Cage free and whole grain or vegetable fed chickens produce eggs with the best nutritional value. Commercial chicken farmers cage chickens and make it so that the chickens are continuously exposed to light both night and day in order to make the chickens produce more eggs –this is not natural. When chickens are provided with quality feed and living conditions, their eggs will be more nutritious for us to eat.

Eggs should be washed thoroughly before they are cracked open. It has recently become more common for people, whether living in a small city or in the country, to raise their own chickens, so, they eat their own organically grown eggs. Regardless of their origin, eggs that are not washed well can become contaminated because bacteria can get through small holes in the eggshell. Also, storing eggs in warmer temperatures can increase the chance of bacteria being able to infiltrate the eggs. It is important to store eggs in the refrigerator, even farm fresh eggs.

Eggs should be eaten only when they have been fully cooked. The best way to eat eggs is to steam, hard-boil or scramble them as these preparations will sterilize the eggs. About 0.2% of Americans are allergic to eggs,[31] so you must be extra cautious when introducing eggs to infants and children. Allergies to eggs can be so severe that even the smell of a cooked egg can cause a reaction. It is generally recommended that children under 12 months not be given egg products (including products that contain eggs, such as egg noodles, some ice creams, etc.).

Supplements

More than half of American adults take at least one dietary supplement.[32] Supplements include vitamins, minerals, antioxidants, protein drinks and bars, weight loss bars, probiotics, fish oil and herbs. Supplements are so popular that they are considered an essential part of the American diet. But, are supplements really good for your health? Supplements can be considered medicinal for people in need of them. Here are a couple of examples.

1. If a person is very ill and unable to eat or digest food well then they will most likely have a nutritional deficiency, in this case supplements are necessary.

2. Some people take diuretics and consequently lose too many minerals through urinating frequently, so they need to take mineral supplements to compensate for the minerals lost through frequent urination.

3. Some people develop a digestive disorder due to an imbalance of good and bad bacteria in their digestive system caused by taking antibiotics. They may choose to take probiotics to help restore the bacteria and yeast balance in their gut.

4. If someone has a low HDL level they may choose to take a fish oil supplement to help raise their HDL level.

However, for persons with normal health, taking supplements everyday might not be helpful, on the contrary, it may actually be harmful. Remember, supplements are medicine, not food. Additionally, supplements are processed and concentrated and may contain harmful additives and preservatives. Taking supplements too often or incorrectly can be toxic. For example, an overdose of vitamin A can damage the liver and can even cause cirrhosis. I heard a story about a mother who learned that vitamin A is good for eyesight, so she purchased supplements and gave her two year old and four year old daughters a daily adult dosage of vitamin A. Two years later her children became severely ill. At the hospital the doctor discovered that both her daughters had developed severe liver cirrhosis. Their livers were so seriously damaged that they both had to have liver transplants in order to survive. All of these health complications occurred because the children were given an adult dosage of vitamin A –clearly these supplements can be toxic.

Supplements place a lot of stress on the liver. When supplements are processed into pills there are many chemicals involved. These chemicals can be potentially lethal to your health. If there is something on the list of ingredients that you do not understand or have never heard of, it is most likely a chemical, which may cause you problems. For example, a patient of mine had Crohn's disease and started taking vitamin and mineral supplements because she was worried she was not absorbing enough nutrients. After taking supplements her Crohn's syndrome worsened. She discovered that the preservatives in the vitamins she was taking caused the worsening of her condition.

There is no research or study that definitively proves that taking extra doses (above the recommended daily limit) of vitamins and minerals can prevent illnesses and diseases, such as the common cold or cancer. Supplements can only be preventative in cases where there is a deficiency. Here are some important questions to ask yourself when you are considering supplementing you diet.

1. What is the purpose of taking a fiber supplement? Fiber is needed to avoid constipation and maintain regular bowel movements. Fiber comes from whole grains and vegetables, so why should you take processed fiber pills? Eating the right foods such as whole grains, vegetables and fruits can provide all the fiber you need.

2. Does it make sense to take a pill to lose weight? Doesn't it make more sense to alter your diet and change your lifestyle to lose weight?

3. Is it necessary to take supplements to avoid catching a cold? Through eating correctly you can maintain your immune system's abilities. Taking pills seems like a faster and easier solution, but the fact of the matter is that these supplements do not work.

4. Should you take pills to maintain healthy cholesterol levels? Does it make more sense to exercise and eat fewer calories in order to achieve healthy cholesterol levels naturally? If you eat properly, your cholesterol will certainly not be high. Again, taking pills seems like a much easier solution, but pills cannot help you achieve real, long-term good health.

Taking pills has become a habitual part of the American culture. Many people place a lot of faith in their pills to the point where if they forget to take them they feel mentally uncomfortable for the rest of the day. My patients are always surprised when I tell them I do not take any pills or supplements. Some of them can't even imagine that it is possible to be healthy without taking supplements. This entire book is about how to live and eat in order to naturally achieve and maintain a healthy body and mind. However, many Americans mistakenly believe that a healthy body and mind can come from taking supplements. It is important to educate yourself (with books like this one) and not just trust supplement advertising and various health companies in order to find out what actually creates true health. You must remember what is in a company's best interest is most likely not what is in your best interest.

Everybody knows that prevention based health care is the best approach to take. Some people wrongly view supplements as preventative medicine. For example, a patient of mine gave her son a multivitamin daily, and yet he continued to catch a cold often. She thought supplements were a means to strengthen his immune system and prevent him from catching a cold. This, quite simply, is not accurate. For example, taking too many antioxidants can interfere with breast cancer therapy.[33] Supplement companies can bend their information and wrongly misinform the general public. Remember that their best interest, i.e. making a profit, is not in your health's best interest.

Supplement companies misguide people with advertisements and manipulate well known information. For example, fiber is good for the digestive system, so they create fiber supplements. Most people know that fiber is important, so they assume that fiber supplements must be beneficial for their health. They are told that fiber is essential for them to maintain good health and then they are convinced that they certainly must not be getting enough fiber; they begin to worry and are handed an immediate solution and told the only reasonable solution to their concern is to supplement. Fiber rich supplements can lead to unpleasant experiences including gas, bloating and other digestive discomforts. In most circumstances, it is better to eat a diet that provides you with the fiber you need.

Here are just a few reasons that explain why supplements are not necessary and sometimes unhealthy and possibly harmful.
Because supplements are highly concentrated it is easy to overdose, which can be stressful on the body. A friend of mine is very health conscious. He takes multivitamins and mineral pills, antioxidants, fish oil and an energy drink in addition to eating one bowl of whole grain, enriched cereal every morning. After his morning supplements and breakfast he feels confident that he has taken every necessary measure to be in good health. However, in addition to his supplements he also eats fruits and vegetables, which are natural sources of vitamins and minerals. He doesn't take into account that he is going to be eating natural vitamin sources throughout the day. He could actually be taxing his body by over supplementing. Most likely the supplements are not necessary for him.

There is no way we can accurately determine or measure how many supplements should be taken. For example, let's say you take a supplemental dose of vitamin D daily. The amount in the supplement may be well over one hundred percent of the daily recommended allowance. Perhaps you want to be extra healthy, so you take two doses. But, if you are consuming dairy, eggs and fish daily and getting plenty of sunshine, you are already getting vitamin D from other sources. The supplement may not be necessary for you. Vitamin D stays in your body for several weeks, so taking too much vitamin D every day may provide your liver with a potentially toxic build up and cause kidney damage as well. Symptoms of vitamin D overdose include grogginess and constipation. It is best to acquire your dietary needs through foods.

We need to stop worrying about nutritional deficiencies. These days, our problem is being over nourished. In the past when food was not as available, nutritional deficiencies were common, but today, in the modern world, overnutrition is a much bigger problem than nutritional deficiencies.

Some people believe that taking vitamins can combat or be an excuse for eating an unhealthy diet (junk food). But this is nonsense. The only way to have a healthy body is to eat a healthy diet. A healthy diet is the best way to supply your body with the nutrition it needs. It is best to know what your particular body needs and what your health demands, and to eat the foods that supply the necessary nutrition. Educate yourself about the different nutritional values of varying foods. For example, we know we need fresh vegetables and fruits to replenish vitamin C in the body and about two or three medium sized oranges contain enough vitamin C for one day. These kinds of food facts enable us to choose to eat the foods that will provide us with the best nutrition for our individual needs.

Research shows that people who take supplements regularly are most likely to be in worse health than people who do not take supplements because supplements contribute to overnutrition. For example, studies show that too much iron can cause premature aging, cancer, osteoporosis, diabetes, arthritis, heart disease, liver damage and severe fatigue.[34]

Supplements should not be considered preventative medicine and are not a shortcut to good health. Yes, it is easier to spend money on pills than to actually devote time to lifestyle change and taking proper care of your health. The best way to be healthy is to study and find out the natural nutrition sources that are best suited to your needs. Create a unique list of foods for your individual needs, taking into consideration your allergies, intolerances, caloric needs and particular health issues that may be addressed through dietary changes. Overall, it is important to study about the foods you eat and become aware of how much to eat, what you should eat and how to prepare your food. This is the best means of prevention and the most necessary investment in your health. There are no shortcuts in health –you must work hard to achieve and maintain a balanced, healthy body.

Water and Fluids

Water is the most important substance for all living creatures. Without water, human beings cannot survive more than a few days. Dehydration causes thirst, dry skin, dry lips and mouth, fatigue and dizziness. Severe dehydration can cause kidney failure and death. Long-term or chronic dehydration can cause dry eyes and skin, constipation, low immune ability, kidney stones, arteriosclerosis and rapid aging. As you age, you will feel less thirsty, so it is important to drink regularly instead of waiting until you feel thirsty. Regardless of whether or not you drink water, the body is constantly losing water through urination, bowel movements, sweating, breathing and evaporation from the surface of the skin. It is absolutely necessary to drink water regularly and eat foods rich in water.

The water you consume is mainly in fluid form, such as water, tea, juice, coffee, soup, etc. However, foods such as fresh fruits and veggies also contain water. Solid foods can produce water after being metabolized. The byproducts of burned glucose are water and carbon dioxide.

The best way to supply your body the water it needs is by drinking water. Spring water and water obtained from underground sources are best. Well water is better than lake or river water because the latter sources are open and can be polluted by bacteria, chemicals and heavy metals. However, if you drink well water, you still need to make sure it is tested every few years for heavy metals and other minerals. This is particularly important if you live near a fault line, underground hot springs or an active volcano area as these factors can alter the water quality. Some ground water may contain too much sulfur, iron and arsenic.

Most public water sources in America are safe to drink because water service providers abide by certain health standards such as testing the mineral, metal and bacterial content of the water. These services filter and decontaminate the water supply pretty effectively. It is still best to drink water that has been boiled, such as in hot tea, soup or simply plain water after it has cooled.

The benefits of boiling water involve the elimination of chlorine, which is added to nearly all city water in order to kill bacteria, make the water sterile and soften the minerals contained in water. Boiling water is a way to sterilize water. Many Asian cultures boil water before drinking it. This is mainly because Asian countries have a cultural habit of not enjoying cold or cool drinks and foods. It is not common, even today, for an area's water system to provide clean drinking water to the people in these countries. Their habit of boiling water has provided them with, at first, the unintentional (and now commonly understood) benefit of protecting themselves from harmful organisms that may be present in the water. For example, in the 1800's Chinese immigrants came to the West to mine for gold and build railroads. Europeans would get sick after drinking creek water, whereas Chinese people did not get sick because they would boil creek water before drinking it. Various animals' habitats are near and in water sources, so animal waste, fungi and bacterium from the forest can contaminate wild water sources. Boiling water eliminates nearly all of these toxins through sterilization.

Is bottled water safe? People drink bottled water because it is assumed that bottled water is safe and is convenient for travel and transit. However, bottled water is not a perfect solution for your water needs. Bottled water is most commonly packed in plastic bottles. Plastic contains carcinogens which can leak into the water, especially when the plastic has been heated by exposure to high temperatures or sunlight.[35, 36] There is no way to know what happens to bottled water during the shipping and storage process. The bottles may sit in harsh sunshine for hours at a time before arriving at the store. I have seen so many cases of bottled water sitting outside of stores during summer months. It may seem convenient and healthy, but consider the amount of toxins being released into the water while it spends days under the hot sun. The only thing you can know is what happens to the bottled water after you have bought it.

When my oldest daughter was born I purchased a gallon of water at the supermarket that was labeled as water safe for infants. When I got home and opened the bottle I could smell the plastic. After smelling such strong plastic I refused to give her this contaminated water. Eight years later, the same bottle and same brand is still being sold in stores labeled as safe for infants. This water is for babies, so it should be the safest water there is, but it is clear that just because water is in a bottle does not mean it is safe.

The quality of bottled water differs from brand to brand. Some bottled water contains no minerals and is, therefore, too soft. Softened water is not healthy to drink and not good for your stomach. Your body needs trace minerals like potassium, sodium and calcium. People who drink water while playing sports and those who have osteoporosis especially need the trace minerals found in non-softened water. Spring water and underground water naturally contain these minerals. Additionally, some bottled water tastes better because it has additives, flavors and added carbonation in the water. Some bottled water is simply city water that has been packaged. This type of water is usually labeled as drinking water, purified water or filtered water. You are basically buying tap water that has been packaged to look more attractive. Facilities that bottle water may not meet food manufacturing standards and the water may arrive to you already contaminated. I have often opened a bottle of water, let it sit for a few hours and have found that when I reopen the bottle, there is a very unpleasant smell coming from the bottle. This is caused by the bacteria present in the water or the packaging. Once any present bacteria have been exposed to air by opening the bottle, they grow rapidly and the water becomes unsafe to drink.

Bottled water is expensive. In some places, bottled water costs more than any other non-alcoholic bottled beverage. I have commonly seen people pay four or five dollars for a liter of special, imported bottled water. It is both cheaper and healthier to simply boil your own tap water from your home. There are appliances available that allow for rapid boiling, however, the ones made of plastic or aluminum should not be used. It is best to store the water you plan to take with you when you leave your home in metal or glass drinking containers. You can find these containers easily. Many glass drinking containers come with a protective sleeve on the outside to reduce the risk of broken glass from dropping the container.

A common question my patients ask me is, "How much water should I drink every day?" The general consensus is that the average adult should drink eight glasses (eight ounces each) of water a day. But, in the same way it is difficult to tell someone how much they should eat, it is nearly impossible to know how much water someone should drink. There is no exact number or answer that fits everyone's needs. The amount of water you should drink depends on some of the following factors.

1. How active are you? You need to drink more water as your activity increases. If you are very active, then you should drink much more water than you drink when you are not active.

2. What is the surrounding temperature? Even drinking as much as two gallons of water while working outdoors in the hot temperatures of summer may not be enough. In cold temperatures less water is lost through sweat and respiration, so less water needs to be replaced.

3. How well does your digestive system work? For example, if you have diarrhea or many bowel movements you are continuously losing water and so it absolutely necessary to drink more water in order to avoid dehydration and kidney failure.

4. What types of food and other beverages do you consume? For example, fruits, such as oranges and watermelon, and vegetables are rich in water; when you eat these foods you fulfill part of your water needs. If you drink soda or alcohol, you need to drink water more water to counteract the dehydrating effects caused by these beverages.

5. What is your current health condition? For example, if you have a serious illness, such as kidney or liver failure, then you need to be cautious and not drink too much or too little water. It is necessary to consult your doctor about how much water you should be drinking in these types of situations.

The amount of water that each person needs is not only based on the above circumstances. There are so many factors that determine how much water a person needs that is ridiculous to say that there is a certain amount of water that everyone should drink every day. The best way to figure out if you drink too much or too little water is not to count or measure how much you drink, but rather to consider how many times you urinate. If you regularly release a full bladder's worth of urine about four to eight times within twenty-four hours, this may be considered normal and most likely you are drinking enough fluids to meet your body's needs. A full bladder is approximately 500 ml or half of a liter (the liquid amount in a regular water bottle). So, about two to four liters of urine should be produced daily. However, if you have kidney stones, then you should be drinking more water to help flush out the stones and uric acid. Certain medications cause you to urinate more often (sometimes up to five times an hour). It is also important that you urinate regularly throughout the day (about once every few hours), as opposed to going often in a short amount of time.

Can drinking water cause health problems? Like anything else, too much water can affect your health. Drinking water in moderation is the key. If you drink too much water in a short period of time, especially after being dehydrated, the water can rush to the brain and cause brain swelling and even death. This happens to some marathon runners[37] and people who participate in water drinking contests.[38]

If you drink too much water before going to sleep, you can seriously affect the quality of your sleep. Getting up to urinate throughout the night is disruptive. Morning is the best time to drink plenty of water, because you most likely have spent about eight hours without drinking any liquids and are inevitably slightly dehydrated. Drinking a lot of water in the morning will help detox your body and combat dehydration throughout the day. Your body will be able to process the fluid while you are awake instead of when you are trying to get a good night's sleep. People who have metabolism problems, such as kidney or liver failure, should be very cautious about how much water they drink and make sure to abide by their doctor's recommendations.

Water Temperature Can Affect Your Health

Hot water (and other hot beverages) can burn or irritate the tongue, esophagus and stomach and can cause inflammation in various organs potentially leading to pharyngitis, gastritis, inflammation of the tongue, nausea and discomfort in the stomach. Also, if you drink hot water frequently, you may find that you get a sore or dry throat often. Hot water is addictive. Some people will only drink hot water, which can damage the stomach. This is why in China, a culture where many people drink hot water and tea often, it is commonly stated that nine out of ten people will have stomach problems at some point in their lives. If you have gastritis or acid reflex, it is best to just drink warm water and beverages.

Drinking room temperature and warm water is best. Drinking water that is too cold can also be unhealthy. In American culture, most people prefer to drink cold, iced water and beverages. Cold water can damage the stomach, cause gastritis and worsen heartburn. A certain percentage of people are sensitive to cold temperatures. Some people's fingers are very sensitive to cold air and water, such as people who have Raynaud's syndrome, and may have severe reactions to exposure to cold (similar to an allergic reaction). Some people with asthma are sensitive to cold air. In the same way that your hands or windpipe can be sensitive or intolerant to cold temperatures, so can your digestive system. People who have cold hands and feet or Raynaud's syndrome should be extra cautious about drinking cold water.

Additionally, cold water numbs the taste buds. So, when you eat greasy foods along with cold beverages, your body does not resist the overconsumption of grease by signaling nausea or digestive discomfort. This allows people to unknowingly over consume unhealthy and greasy (high fat) foods. This overconsumption causes a person to eat more calories than their body needs and is a contributing factor to weight gain.

Other ways water temperature can affect your health. Drinking cold water in hot weather or after playing sports may cause stomach cramps. Drinking extremely hot and cold liquids together can damage your teeth. Drinking or eating something hot and following it immediately with a cold liquid can cause you to experience toothaches.

Some people recommend drinking fluids or soups before eating in order to fill the belly and help with weight loss. Also, it is common in most cultures to drink soup before the main meal. If you are not trying to lose weight, it is best to avoid drinking a large amount of water before a meal because doing so hinders the abilities of stomach acid. Stomach acid is absolutely necessary for breaking down and absorbing minerals. Stomach acid is also a natural defense system by making food sterile by killing bacteria and other germs. So, in order to give your stomach acid enough time to begin breaking down the food, it is better to drink a small amount of water at least thirty minutes or more after a meal. This is especially important for people who have acid reflex. It is important to drink water and fluids regularly throughout the day. It is not a good idea to drink a lot of water once or twice a day.

If you are experiencing bouts of diarrhea, loss of blood, menstruation, kidney stones, body aches and pains or if you have gout, it is important to drink more water throughout the day in order to prevent dehydration. Water is the best way to detox (cleanse) your body.

Some medications are very toxic, so it is important to drink plenty of water as a means to thin the concentration of the medication in your body and assist your stomach in absorbing it better. This will reduce your chance of getting medicine-related organ irritation. If you take diuretic pills, you will become dehydrated easily because you urinate more frequently. How much to drink depends on your health condition and you should talk to your doctor about this. However, do not blindly trust your doctor. Diuretics are often prescribed as quick fixes. For example, older people who have leg edema may retain water because of inactivity or arteriosclerosis, which prevents fluids from flowing properly throughout the body. If given a diuretic, these people will become dehydrated, which is bad for their kidneys. It is better to address the cause of leg edema and pursue alternative treatment rather than taking diuretic pills.

Soda

Another common fluid people consume is soda. Most people know that soda is not a healthy drink, but soda remains a popular and heavily consumed drink. Soda is addictive because of all the sugar, caffeine and additives it contains. These ingredients make people crave the taste of soda. Many people think that drinking diet soda is healthier than regular soda, but most diet sodas use artificial sugars that increase your cravings for it, which will cause you to drink more soda, thereby causing you to ingest more unhealthy chemicals and additives. In short, diet soda is not healthier than regular soda and may actually be more harmful. Sweeteners in soda, regardless of their origin, can irritate the stomach and are known to commonly cause heartburn when over consumed. If you are already suffering from heartburn, it is likely that drinking soda will make your condition worse.

The majority of sodas contain additives such as cane sugar, corn syrup, sodium, colorings and caffeine. Drinking soda regularly can make water seem plain and boring, so soda becomes the drink of choice. Soda makes people hyper, so drinking it late at night or before going to bed can keep you awake and affect the quality of your sleep. In addition, soda contains calories, but, because it is a liquid, many people do not consider just how many calories they have drunk and do not adjust their food intake to prevent the overconsumption of calories. If you have a weight problem, do not forget to count soda calories. If you have high blood pressure and are worried about salt intake, then you have to make sure to count the sodium intake in any soda you may drink as well.

Coffee

Another common beverage is coffee. It is one of the most common drinks in America. Coffee is the result of burning coffee beans and then running very hot water through them. Regular coffee beans are actually a light, milky green color. Coffee beans bought from the store are brown or black because they have been roasted until burnt. As discussed earlier, burnt food contains a high percentage of cancer causing carcinogens, so drinking too much coffee may cause health issues.

The majority of people who drink coffee do so because they are addicted to it. Coffee contains caffeine, an addictive substance, and is often drunk while hot (the temperature excites the taste buds). Some people are so addicted that if they do not drink coffee for even one day they will experience withdrawal symptoms that often involve painful headaches, fatigue and inability to concentrate. People often add sugar and milk to coffee because very few people like the taste of black coffee, but these additives actually make coffee more addictive. In fact, many people like the sweetness of the sugar and greasiness of the cream more than they actually like coffee. Many people drink coffee because they feel coffee gives them an energy boost and can help them feel awake and alert. But, when you are tired it is important to treat it properly by getting more sleep, exercise and proper nourishment, instead of a quick, unnecessary fix like coffee. Coffee may be considered unhealthy because:

1. Roasted coffee is a burnt food, and in my opinion, poses similar risks as eating other types of burnt foods.

2. Sugar and cream added to coffee adds unnecessary calories to your diet and may increase your cravings for it.

3. Coffee is addictive.[39]

4. The caffeine in coffee can cause health problems, such as increased sweating and increase your chance of developing high blood pressure.[40]

5. Coffee is highly acidic. The acid can bind to calcium and eventually cause a kidney stone. If you already have kidney stones or have had kidney stones, you should use caution and make sure to drink weaker coffee and more water.[41]

4. Don't drink coffee that is stored or bottled in certain plastics or metal cans because these containers may contain BPA which has been linked to health ailments.[42]

5. Coffee is one of the most pesticide laden foods on the market today. Drinking pesticides probably negates any claimed benefits of drinking coffee.[43]

Teas

There are many different types of tea including black tea, green tea, herbal tea, etc. In recent years, there have been many reports explaining how green tea can be beneficial to your health. Claims that the antioxidants in green tea can slow down the aging and hardening of your arteries, reduce your chance of having a heart attack and can prevent or reduce the chance of urinary tract infection and bladder cancer have been made. Although green tea does contain antioxidants, the amount does not surpass the amount of antioxidants in fresh fruits and vegetables.[44] The reason why green tea can reduce many health risks is likely caused by the fact that when drinking green tea you are also drinking water. Water will flush toxic uric acid out of your body which will prevent the uric acid from irritating or damaging your arteries. Not all teas are beneficial for your health. Here a few guidelines to take into consideration when adding tea to your diet.

1. Avoid drinking green tea that is too concentrated. Green tea is acidic and does contain caffeine, so when it is too strong it can increase your chance of developing a kidney stone.

2. Tea bags can be unhealthy because they contain often contain wax, mold, chlorine and other chemicals that can leak into the tea. Tea bags are not usually packed airtight, so it is easier for mold to develop. Moldy tea is toxic for the body. Therefore, loose tea is much better for your health. In China, where green tea originated, people rarely use tea bags. Tea bags are commonly bleached as a means to inhibit mold and bacteria growth. When the tea bag is exposed to hot water, these toxins are released into the tea. Adding bleach to your diet may very well counteract the intended benefits of drinking tea.

3. Do not drink green tea in the form of sodas or bottled drinks. These drinks contain a lot of sugar and corn syrup and pose similar health risks as soda.

4. Don't drink tea that is stored and bottled in aluminum cans. Aluminum cans are coated with BPA and aluminum itself can be toxic.[45]

5. Do not add sugar or cream to green tea because this can increase your cravings for it.

6. When green tea is processed into black tea (through a process that is similar to fermentation) some toxic chemicals are produced. The topic as to which type of tea is healthiest is widely debated and I, personally, have not concluded which teas are or are not healthier to consume.

7. Since it was discovered that green tea may be good for your health, many green tea products have been marketed to the public, such as green tea soda, drinks, pills, powder, ice cream, extracts, shampoo, lotions, etc. I doubt these products provide any substantial health benefits.

8. Recently, it has been discovered that many teas being imported from China contain high levels of banned pesticides and herbicides.[46] Certainly, any potential health benefits of drinking tea would be lost by consuming these toxic additives. It is best to only drink organic teas and to purchase them only from reputable companies who have met strict standards. It isn't enough to simply trust the label of a product, you should be able to verify the company has met the requirements it claims.

10. As with other drinks, it is quite possible that many of the health benefits derived from drinking all of the different kinds of teas may simply be the addition of water to your diet.

Herbal Tea

Herbs have been regarded as medicine in Chinese and almost all other cultures for centuries. However, nowadays in America, herbs are considered to be supplements that should be added to our daily diet – but herbs are powerful medicines. Many synthetic drugs are manmade replicas of herbs and herbal folk remedies. It is commonly known that aspirin originated from willow tree bark. When taking prescriptions you should be very careful about drinking herbal tea because an improper combination may cause complications and lead to severe health problems. If taking herbs, you should abide by the recommendations of a properly trained herbalist. If you want to make your own herbal teas, then you should educate yourself about the various types of herbs and make sure to avoid negative combinations. For example, ginger tea is popularly used in Chinese medicine as aspirin. Ginger tea can relieve a sore throat, nausea, thin blood to release pain and prevent blood clots; the blood thinning capacities of ginger tea can be beneficial for people who suffer from cold hands and feet. However, if you take blood thinning medication in combination with drinking ginger tea, your blood might be thinned out too much. Additionally, many people have reactions to some herbs; if you feel discomfort or any other type of reaction to herbal tea, then you should stop drinking it immediately. Again, whenever possible, consume only organic herbal teas in order to avoid a highly concentrated dose of chemicals.

Soup

Broth based soups are rich in water and flavor and are one of the healthiest foods you can eat. Different cultures have different kinds of soup. Soup can make you full, provide you with plenty of water and can prevent you from eating too many calories by naturally lowering your appetite. But, of course, soup is not perfect. Here are some points to keep in mind about soup.

1. Soup is liquid. We drink it; we don't need to chew it much, if at all. So, it provides less stimulation to the digestive system. Eating soup regularly for a long time can cut down your appetite and can lead to the development of food intolerances. People with poor digestion or a digestive disorder, such as IBS, Crohn's disease, colitis, etc. should avoid drinking soup often. If you have discomfort in your belly, drinking soup can give your digestive system a rest, but a long-term soup diet can cause digestive disorders because drinking soup does not fully exercise your digestive tract.

2. When cooking soup, you should make sure to focus on nutrition more than flavor. It is important to measure the ingredients, especially if you add sugar or salt, instead of adding a lot for the sake of flavor. Soup is mostly water. Water thins out salt and sugar, so adding salt and sugar for the sake of taste will often lead you to add too much. Try using different spices to add sodium-free flavor to the soups you make.

3. Do not overcook vegetables when making soup. Cooking vegetables with meat can diminish the nutritional value of vegetables. If you are making soup that contains meat, then make sure to cook the meat first, and later, when the meat is nearly done, add the vegetables.

4. Do not eat soup when it is very hot. Hot liquids can burn the tongue, throat and esophagus. Hot liquids may damage your stomach and may cause pharyngitis and tonsillitis. Drinking soup that is so hot that it makes you sweat is not healthy. People think that drinking hot soup will help them to battle a cold, but it will merely cause internal damage. Drink soup that is warm.

5. It is best to avoid using canned soup because it is can increase your risk of cancer and heart disease because the lining in cans contain harmful chemicals that leak into the soup.[47] Use extra caution when buying packaged soup. Soup mixes that have been packaged in plastic or paper and prepared soups that have been packaged in plastic or glass may contain additives and preservatives, just look at the list of

ingredients and you will see the various chemicals that have been added to the soup in order to prolong its shelf life or add to its flavor. Soups that are heated and served hot in plastics may absorb more toxins than unheated soups that are stored in these types of containers.[48] If you want to eat soup at a restaurant, be sure to ask if the soup is heated or held in plastic lined crock pots or steam pans and if so, do not order it. Don't use plastic containers to heat soup in the microwave. Making your own soup is much healthier.

How to Prepare and Cook Your Food for Better Health

Cooking can make food taste better, easier to digest, reduce food intolerance and sterilize food. However, if it is not cooked correctly, even the healthiest food can become damaging to your health. Cooking foods at too high of a temperature can damage the nutritional value of your food, burnt food can produce carcinogens and cooking food for too long or incorrectly can produce toxic byproducts.[49] There are simple ways to reduce your risk of compromising your health by changing the way you prepare food.

Raw Foods –some foods can be eaten raw, for example most fruits and vegetables. Raw foods usually provide a better source of nutrition than cooked foods. However, eating raw food is not always healthy or practical. Raw foods may be contaminated with parasites, bacteria and other germs. If cooked, foods can be sterilized; therefore effectively killing potentially deadly bacteria such as E.coli and salmonella.[50] Meat and fish can be very parasitic as a result of coming into contact with, eating or drinking contaminated food and water sources (while it is alive). For many people eating vegetables, both cooked and raw, is somewhat of a chore.

Raw vegetables tend to be less tasty than cooked vegetables. When we cook vegetables flavor can be infused into them, thereby making them more acceptable to children and pickier eaters. Many people are repulsed by the idea of eating raw fish, but fish can become quite appetizing to these people after it has been seasoned and cooked.

Eating raw food can increase your chances of developing a food intolerance or food allergy and general discomfort from bloating, gas, cramps or acid reflex. When cooked, food is better tolerated by your digestive system. Some foods, such as soybeans, can be toxic if eaten raw or undercooked. In some Asian cultures, soybeans are the main protein source. If eaten raw, soybeans can cause serious problems such as swelling of the pancreas. Most fruits can be eaten raw and some foods are best when eaten raw such as cucumbers, radishes and lettuce. However, if you have a digestive disorder, such as IBS or acid reflex, or have a weakened digestive system (common in ill or elderly persons) cooked vegetables are easier for your belly to handle.

Boiling and Poaching –boiling is one of the best ways to cook food. Boiling temperature is 212 degrees Fahrenheit. This temperature is hot enough to kill nearly all germs and parasites, thereby sterilizing food and making it safe to eat. Boiling both sterilizes and softens water and can remove chlorine from water. Boiling can fully cook food without burning it and is a great way to infuse various levels of flavor into what is being cooked. Boiling is the best way to cook whole grains and beans, because it breaks down fiber, making the food easier to digest. Boiling creates the least pollution in your home. Steam does not produce strong odors, unlike grilling and baking.

Like anything else, boiling food does have some negative aspects. Boiling food for too long can destroy the nutritional value of food, such as precious vitamins. Vegetables should not be boiled for too long. It is easy to consume too much salt or sugar when it is added to boiling water (as when making soups). Boiling water and food can be dangerous, so make sure to supervise children when they are around anything that is cooking or is still hot from having been cooked.

Steaming Food –steaming creates about the same cooking temperature as boiling and is a similar way to prepare food that uses less water than boiling. Steaming is the best way to cook bread. Bread can be fully cooked without becoming crispy or burnt on the surface. Also, steaming bread makes it softer, which makes it easier to chew and gentler on the throat. Fish and rice can be fully cooked through steaming without being burnt. When vegetables are steamed they lose less nutrition than when they are boiled. Steam also creates less pollution in your home.

Baking –baking can be a healthy way to cook food, especially if the baking temperature is not set too high. Broiling is a form of baking at high temperatures and should be avoided. Most people bake food for too long at temperatures that are too high, which can burn food. The most common example of this is bread that has very dark crust. Bread

that is browned (burnt) contains carcinogens that are toxic.[51]
Additionally, if bread is baked at too high of a temperature the outside
will cook faster and cause the inside to be undercooked. Eating the
undercooked portion of the bread can lead to food intolerance. Baking
can create pollution your home. Cleaning the oven with high
temperatures burns leftover grease and oil that pollutes the home and
can be bad for those who have respiratory disorders. In the kitchen,
baking is the main cause of skin burns.

Stir-frying –stir-frying is a light frying and is a healthy way to cook.
Stir-frying originated in China. The Chinese culture has a history of
over five thousand years, so there has been plenty of time to develop
effective and healthy ways to eat and cook. Stir-frying has remained the
most popular form of healthy cooking in Asia and is popular in other
countries. But stir-frying must be done properly. When done correctly,
stir-frying is one of the best ways to flavor vegetables. The proper way
to stir-fry is to put a couple tablespoons of oil in a pan and wait for the
oil to heat up. Then put thinly sliced pieces of meat and onions or
garlic or other seasonings in the oil and add some water to prevent
burning. Use a wood or metal spatula to move the meat around
constantly as a way to prevent burning, over cooking and sticking.
After the meat has fully cooked, add the vegetables and mix them for
one to two minutes and eat your stir-fried meal immediately. Always
wash vegetables before cooking them.

Adding flavorings and herbs will make food tastier and, in some cases,
easier to digest. But, some people add too many or unhealthy flavor
enhancers, like MSG, processed soybean products, chicken broth and
salt, all of which can be very unhealthy when used in any quantity (for
those who are intolerant or allergic to them) or when overused.
Concern for your health should come first –not flavor. For example,
artificial sweeteners can be very toxic. One mother in China would
make stir-fried eggs with sugar for her daughter because it was the only
way her daughter would eat eggs and her mother believed that it was
necessary for her daughter to eat eggs in order to get enough protein.
One day the mother ran out of sugar and used an artificial sweetener
instead. The mother did not know that when this artificial sweetener
was heated it became toxic. Unfortunately her daughter had a severe
reaction to the toxin and died. How tragic to have to die from flavoring
food.

Although stir-frying, when done properly, is healthy; it is still considered frying. The smoke produced from heating the oil, the heating of spices, sauces, onions, peppers and garlic can create air pollution inside your home. Always use proper ventilation when cooking by using fans that exhaust outside of your home or open a window or door in your home to remove the smoke and odors created from cooking.

Pan Frying –pan frying or sautéing is not considered as healthy as stir-frying because people tend to use too much oil when frying this way. It is easy to overheat the oil and burn food when pan frying which also creates pollution in your home.

Deep Fat Frying –deep frying is used to cook meat, potatoes, breaded vegetables and meats, etc. The most famous foods in America include fried chicken and french-fries. If hot enough, the oil from deep frying will burn any type of food. A lot of carcinogens are able to accumulate in oil because the oil tends to be used many times before being changed. This is why in recent years standards have been developed in order to avoid the creation of too many carcinogens.[52] However, it can be difficult to know when a new batch of oil should be used. Plus, not every restaurant follows these guidelines; so it is best for you to assume that fried food that has not been cooked by you has either been cooked in toxic oil or has been fried for too long. Generally speaking, although fried food is tasty, it is very unhealthy. In fact, deep fat frying is the unhealthiest way to prepare any type of food.

Any frying method done at very high temperatures can be dangerous and unhealthy. For example, in some Asian restaurants, it is common for the cooks to heat up cooking oil until it smokes (caused by the oil burning) and then stir-fry the meats, eggs or vegetables. This is a very unhealthy way to fry (cook) foods.

Grilling –grilling is one of the most popular ways to cook meat in America. People use burning wood, coal, charcoal, gasoline and propane to grill. During the grilling process food comes into direct contact with smoke and fire, which increases the chance of food becoming burnt. Unfortunately, many Americans greatly enjoy the flavor of burnt meat. Burnt food is unhealthy because it contains carcinogens.[53] Additionally, when grilling, the external color may lead you to believe that the food is done, but it still may be undercooked inside. The distinctive grilled flavor comes from the mix of burnt grease and the substance that is being used to grill (coal, wood, gasoline, etc.). Indeed, grilling is considered a form of art in the United States as people devote much of their time to discovering which types of woods and smoking methods create the best flavors. Although grilled food is indeed very tasty; it is extremely toxic and loaded with carcinogens. Grilled (burnt and smoked) food is one of the top culprits for life-style related cancers.[54, 55] Stomach, colon, pancreatic and several other types of cancers have been linked to carcinogens that are caused by eating too much grilled (burnt and smoked) meat.[56] Eating grilled meat on a daily basis can seriously affect your ability to maintain your health. I have a patient whose husband died at a young age of pancreatic cancer. She told me that her husband only ate organic lean meat and vegetables, but when I asked her how her husband prepared his food she explained that he mainly used the grill.

Smoked Foods –smoked meats and seafood are the most popular types of smoked foods eaten in America. Smoked food creates a taste similar to grilled food. Smoked food is produced by the accumulation of smoke in a closed space or by adding artificial smoke flavor. You would never stand in a room full of smoke because you know that it would be dangerous for your health and difficult to breathe in such an environment. Eating food that has been prepared in such an environment is surely not healthy. Food that is otherwise healthy can become toxic when exposed to unhealthy additives. For example, a patient of mine hunts and fishes for his own meat. The source is healthy, but he processes the meat through grilling and smoking, so it loses its organic health value. When preparing food to be smoked, people often add too much salt and salt rich marinade. Jerked meats often contain artificial smoke flavor and extremely unhealthy levels of salt and other additives, such as MSG.

Use Your Senses to Improve the Quality of Your Diet

We should use common sense and our perceptions to determine what foods are best for us to eat. Your sense of smell can help you determine whether or not a food has rotted. If you find that smoke or odors created from a specific cooking technique are hard to tolerate, such as grilling or smoking foods, then that food is probably toxic. (That is why people always grill outdoors.) You can use your eyes to select the healthiest food. For example, you can clearly see if a food is burnt or has molded or rotted. Your sense of touch and taste can determine whether or not the food is too hot, too spicy or still fresh.

However, food can taste good and not necessarily be good for you. We tend to rely solely on our mouths to determine what to eat. Unfortunately, the unhealthiest food usually tends to taste very good. Because tasty foods are usually high in calories, it is instinctual for us to want to eat these foods.

The most important organ to count on when eating is your brain. You need to think and use the knowledge you already have about various foods in order to make healthy eating decisions. Food can taste good and look good, but only your brain can determine whether or not the food is actually healthy for you. Ingredients, nutritional information, how long food has been stored, where the food comes from, how it has been prepared and packaged and the likelihood that there are bacteria in the food are all things that only your brain can determine.

Use your brain to analyze and make your decisions about what and how much to eat. The more you learn about food, diet and cooking the more knowledge you will have, therefore, you will make healthier and better food choices. However, the brain is a complicated organ, sometimes you may think you are eating what you need or making the right choices, but these choices can be very toxic to your health. Understanding the relationship between food and mental health is complex, but it is crucial to understand this relationship in order to be able to eat and live well.

Food and Mental Well-being

Our behavior is very much a product of our mind. Eating, like other activities, is a behavior that can become a form of health abuse. However, unlike other destructive activities such as excessive use of alcohol, smoking and drugs; overeating is not considered morally or ethically wrong because it does not cause explicit harm to other individuals. So, there are no external laws to combat overeating. But, eating is the number one cause of most diseases in America, and causes more deaths than smoking, drinking and drugs combined.[57] So, regardless of the fact that no laws exist to stop us from overeating, we should still take the health risks it carries seriously.

The majority of people who overeat do not fully understand that food can cause health problems and that eating habits are intimately tied to the status of their health. (For example, most people do not realize that overeating can cause them to develop metabolic syndrome.) Many people simply do not know how to understand and use the calorie and nutritional information of varying foods to guide them in making food choices that are best for their own specific health needs. You should learn how to eat and what to eat instead of claiming to be uninformed about the subject.

Some people know what and how much they should eat, but do not take it seriously. These are the people who claim, "You only live once." "You cannot take life that seriously." Or, "You should enjoy life!" Just because you might enjoy alcohol doesn't mean you have an excuse to become an alcoholic. The same is true for food. In reality, these people lack willpower. At times we know what our bodies want to eat, but we also know that we shouldn't eat it –plenty of people can make the decision to abstain from these unhealthy food choices and so can you.

A mentality from the past still reigns over our ideas –that is the misconception that as Americans we are not getting enough nutrition from our diets. Before modern times, many foods were scarce; this caused various vitamins and minerals deficiencies in most people's diets. However, the majority of people today do not lack nutrition. In actuality, being overnourished is far more prevalent and causes many more problems than nutritional deficiencies in America today. Therefore, we need to make a shift in our mentality and stop worrying about nutritional deficiencies and focus on proper eating habits and making better food choices.

Many people see eating as pleasurable and entertaining. Food is especially pleasurable when we are actually hungry. Unfortunately, because food has become such a predominant part of our culture, many people eat when they are not hungry. (I wouldn't be surprised if few Americans even know what true hunger feels like.) Eating as a way to pursue pleasure and entertainment as opposed to satisfying physical hunger is a very unhealthy habit and eventually leads to horrible health complications. When we take advantage of eating, it can become a form of self-abuse and or even suicidal-type behavior.

There are ways for you to discipline yourself and develop a new perspective on food; one that divorces itself from the commonly held view that food is a form of entertainment.

1. Most tasty foods are highly addictive. Heavily seasoned, spicy, sweet, bitter, greasy and salty foods are addictive. The most common types of

these foods in our culture are sweet, greasy and salty foods. All of these types of foods are usually high calorie foods as well. In some ways, it is a survival mechanism to eat these calorie dense foods. When eaten moderately, these foods should pose few health problems. These high calorie foods are dangerous, not because they are necessarily bad for you, but because it is extremely easy to overeat these foods. Although some healthy foods do not taste good when you first try them, you can easily develop a liking for them. For example, most people do not like the taste of wine or beer when they first try it, but rather, they learn to like it, enjoy it and even crave it because of the feelings that they experience or associate with drinking these beverages. Another example of a food that is easy to acquire a taste for is spicy food. At first, we can usually only handle mild spices, but the more we eat these spices, the higher tolerance we develop for them. Sometimes our taste buds may be trained to enjoy or even crave spicier foods.

2. Do not simply trust your taste buds. If you simply only use your mouth to choose what you eat, then you will definitely overeat. You need to use your brain, that is, your ability to think and reason, to help discipline your personal eating habits. People may be intolerant or allergic to certain foods that they find very tasty. They may not have an immediate reaction, so they don't immediately associate their health problem with the food they have eaten. But, clearly, regardless of how good a certain food tastes, if you are intolerant or allergic to it, then you should abstain from eating it. It is evident that you cannot just trust your taste buds when it comes to health. It just so happens that food allergy and intolerance reactions are such miserable and uncomfortable experiences most people do not struggle with cutting problem foods completely out of their diets.

3. Your food consumption habits are influenced by the eating habits of those in your immediate environment. This explains why families, as opposed to just one member of the family, tend to be obese or overweight. Like health, life habits can be hereditary. If a man grows up often eating meat and rarely eating vegetables, then when he is forced to change his diet, eating vegetables might bring such displeasure to him that he may experience depression from his dietary changes. Some people who never drink soda will feel that drinking it is torture, whereas people who have been drinking soda since they were a child may find it comforting and very enjoyable. They may even feel that they are missing an important part of their day if they deny themselves their daily soda. Your environment can and does affect how you view food, especially in families or social circles that use food to comfort,

reward, entertain, relax, etc. These habits can be nearly impossible to break in adulthood, especially if you are not honest with yourself about how your views of food were shaped during your childhood and the people you live with now.

4. Social situations can also influence your diet. Similar to social smokers and social drinkers, there is such a thing as being a social eater. Some people get together only to eat or use eating as their only reason to socialize with others. These activities are the result of unconsciously trying to fit into a group. These social situations give food its peak value by providing a form of entertainment that all can enjoy. Food centered gatherings rarely leave anyone feeling left out. It is okay to enjoy these kinds of gatherings. Eating high calorie, commercially prepared meals or eating a large amount of calorie dense foods that are commonly served at social functions is okay once in a while. This becomes a problem only when it eating to socialize becomes a habit or a frequent and normal part of your life. When in a group, it may sometimes seem strange or neurotic to choose healthy foods, so people will often make unhealthy, calorie rich food choices as a way to fit in and participate fully in the social gathering.

5. Your culture influences your personal eating habits. Depending on where and how you are raised, you will eat and not eat certain types of food. For example, Asian cultures tend to steam, boil and stir-fry their food, whereas the American culture prefers grilling, frying and baking. When I tell my patients that I mainly boil the meat that I eat, they are always surprised. It is difficult for them to accept the food practices of other cultures. Cultural practices are constantly changing. For example, baked ham and turkey used to be something that people ate only for special occasions. Now, it is common to find these foods being eaten frequently. Even in China, where turkey is not a native bird, it has become a luxury food item because it is associated with the American lifestyle. Unfortunately, the eating habits of the culture we live in tend to be in response to what tastes good to us, not what is good for our health. It may be unreasonable to think that we will be able to change the culture, but we can take responsibility for ourselves and choose the parts of our culture that we like and make our own style of living and eating. For example, in America we tend to eat an appetizer, main course and then a dessert. We eat salad first, the food that gives us the least pleasure. We then eat some sort of greasy meat dish as the main meal and finally eat a high calorie, sweet food to end the meal on a pleasurable and memorable note. It would be much harder to eat and

enjoy our meal if we were to eat sweet foods first and then salad because low calorie foods are not as tasty as high calorie foods.

6. Eat to live, do not live to eat. You should eat what is healthy for you, not just what gives you pleasure. Some people eat snacks, the most popular of which are candy bars, cookies, crackers, cheese and chips. When people eat snacks they are not actually hungry; they have just developed eating snacks as a hobby. Some people eat snacks that are so high in calories that they end up consuming more calories from snacking then they eat during their actual meals.

7. Using food for comfort and to suppress emotional issues is very common in this country. We can see the origin of this in infants; when a baby is crying we give them something they can eat, drink or keep in their mouths in order to calm themselves. Because eating is pleasurable, it can make us feel happier. But, in excess, food can actually be the cause of health and mental problems.

Overall, use your determination as a tool to help you eat what your body needs instead of what you want to eat. Eating for health is an easy way to achieve a healthy mental attitude towards eating and may help you overcome any eating problems you may be currently facing.

Chapter Three

Exercise and Sports
Why Exercise Can Either
Help or Harm You

How can we stay healthy and prevent diseases? Most people will likely answer, "By eating a healthy diet and exercising regularly." This may be true, but there is a lot of important information about exercise that you need to know in order to properly benefit from it. For example, regular, proper exercise or physical labor is very important for your health and is just as important as what you eat. Improper exercise can wear down your joints, damage your organs, injure your body and can even cause disability or death. Our modern lifestyle includes little physical labor. Therefore, basic movements and exercise are not integrated into many people's lives. Because of this decrease in physical labor, most physical injuries are not the result of labor, but rather from exercise. The majority of these injuries are caused when a person chooses the wrong type of exercise for their individual health needs. If you educate yourself on how to properly exercise based on your unique needs, you can avoid serious injuries.

Your Motivation to Exercise Should Be Health Driven

You should exercise for the betterment of life, not live in order to exercise. The motivation to exercise should be mainly for your health, but unfortunately, there are many unhealthy sources of motivation to exercise, which can in turn damage your health.

Common Reasons People Exercise

Addiction to exercise (sometimes referred to as "runner's high") – some people are addicted to the emotional feeling that they get from intense exercise. Exercise can be addictive, especially extreme sports, because endorphins are released when you exercise. In fact, I am one of many people who are addicted to the satisfying feeling that comes when playing strenuous sports. I began playing basketball when I was ten years old. At first, it was boring and difficult for me, but as I became a teenager I grew to like the game. I went on to play for my college basketball team. I had been enjoying the game for many years and eventually realized that I was addicted to it. Every time I played I felt relaxed, my mind was clearer, I had more energy, I felt a sense of satisfaction, had less pain in my body and experienced emotional and physical feelings of well-being. I enjoyed the game while I was playing it, but if I did not play the game I would crave it. By the time I was thirty-five I had to stop playing basketball regularly or aggressively due to a knee injury. I still miss playing basketball every day. (Even though my knee injury has healed, I avoid playing basketball in order to prevent potential re-injury.)

A patient of mine developed a knee injury due to aggressively playing tennis for over 30 years. I asked her to stop playing tennis and she told me she would rather have her knee replaced than stop playing tennis. When you are willing to put your health at risk, or even deliberately injure yourself, for the sake of a game, you have a sports addiction. Although exercise is good for your health, both physically and emotionally, it can also have the potential to create more damage than benefit for you if you do not engaged in it properly. We should be wise and control our dependency on a sport by cutting down how often we play or taking up a different sport that causes us less injury. If you pursue a sport and disregard the fact that it jeopardizes your health then you have an unhealthy dependency on it, which means you actually have an unhealthy motivation for exercising.

Using exercise to gain attention –some people exercise as a way to "show-off" their physical bodies. Many men lift weights to "bulk up" and some even use steroids (a drug that has a whole slew of unhealthy physical and emotional side effects[1]) in order to "pump up" their muscles. For some, the motivation behind this activity is the notion that big muscles make men look more masculine and attractive to women, but at some point enlarged muscles can actually jeopardize good health. Some men begin weightlifting with reasonable muscle mass goals, but their mental or physical addiction to weightlifting can cause them to not only exceed their initial muscle building goals but to create extreme ideas of the body and strength they want to build. Some people spend a lot of money on expensive equipment or gym memberships, supplements and even traveling to competitions. Some people use exercise as a way to gain attention through social media or blogging by reporting how much weight they lifted, how far they ran or even how much weight they've lost or intend to lose. The motivation behind these postings is usually to gain the praise of their peers and draw attention to their physical accomplishments.

Gyms are breeding grounds for all types of germ infestations because people sweat a lot and share equipment and, in most cases, the air quality in a gym is extremely poor due to lack of proper building ventilation. Gyms try to stay clean by using chemically based disinfectants, but these can also be detrimental to your health. Proper exercise does not require us to spend a lot of money. But with an unhealthy motive, like showing-off, exercising can suddenly become a very expensive endeavor.

Need to compete to gain recognition or reward –some people train for athletic competitions as their life's work, which can push their bodies beyond normal, healthy physical limits. One day, someone asked me if Olympians are healthy. I answered that competing in the Olympic Games is not for health, but rather for reward and title. There are hundreds of thousands of people who practice every day and work hard to reach the goal of being qualified to compete in the Olympic Games. Very few people successfully reach this goal. Many are injured and have to quit practicing because of this and some even become disabled. The prestige and potential rewards that come from competing at the Olympic Games can be a motivating factor for those who train for the Olympics. The fact of the matter is that most professional athletes are motivated to play sports because of some type of expected reward from doing so. Whether to impress someone, perhaps a family or team member, to be named the winner, to receive recognition, to gain material rewards, etc.; these are all forms of reward that motivate people to compete in sports. We even see the role rewards can play in sports in the language used to applaud good goals. For example, I heard a teenager cheer, "Good job, that is money!" when his friend made a good shot during a basketball game. Clearly, playing well is associated with winning and succeeding, which eventually translates into money or some type of reward, such as an MVP title or trophy. Language plays a big role in the way we play sports. For example, a common expression heard from coaches during practice is, "No pain, no gain." From a young age we hear and, therefore, think that part of being good at sports is pushing ourselves and only stopping when we are forced to stop because of physical injury. This mentality exists in the professional sports world where many paid professional football players must live with pain as the result of a sports injury, even after they have retired. Clearly, money in combination with sports can be a dangerous, unhealthy motivation for exercise that can push you beyond what your body can handle.

Exercise and Reproductive Health

Physical exercise can affect your sex hormones, the blood circulation of your reproductive organs and even fertility. Exercise affects the sexual health of men and women differently.

Extreme sports can have an effect on female hormones, which is why women who play professional sports have high percentage of menstrual pain, irregular menstruation and infertility.[2] It is better for women who want to maintain good health to avoid extreme and aggressive physical sports training.

However, regular and proper physical exercise is very important for maintaining the health of the female reproductive organs, especially for women who work at a desk or have jobs that require little physical activity. The female reproductive organs are located at the bottom of the pelvis and because of gravity blood circulation can become static around these organs. This can cause menstrual disorders, fibroids, ovarian cysts, etc. Regular exercise can treat or prevent these types of problems.[3] Regular and proper exercise can strengthen a pregnant woman's abdominal muscles, which can lead to a healthier pregnancy and an easier child birthing experience.[4]

Cardiovascular exercise (jogging, playing tennis, low-impact aerobics or any activity that can adequately raise your heart rate and create sweat) can effectively relieve PMS (premenstrual syndrome). You do not need to exercise for long periods of time; thirty minutes twice a week is sufficient to maintain good menstrual health. Exercise can maintain strong bones. Low-impact exercise, such as walking, is one of the best ways to prevent and treat osteoporosis which affects many older women.

Physical exercise for men, especially extreme competitive sports, can relieve stress. Because of male hormones (such as testosterone), men are more prone to react to stress through anger, irritation, aggression and violence. Playing sports may assist in exhausting stress induced behaviors. It is extremely helpful for teenagers to participate in social sports. These activities can help them regulate their moods as they experience hormonal changes.

Regular physical exercise is important for male reproductive organs, especially for those who work at a desk or in a job that requires little physical activity. Due to gravity, sitting for extended periods of time can cause prostatitis, enlarged prostate, prostate and testicle cancer, varicose veins around the prostate and in the penis, and can reduce libido. Regular exercise can prevent and treat these types of health problems in men.[5]

Men must use extra caution to protect their male reproductive organs while playing extreme sports. Because the majority of male reproductive organs are external to the body, they are more likely to get injured. Injuries may increase the risk of developing cancer.[6] Sometimes the gear and uniform used in a sport can increase the chance of developing testicle and prostate cancer. For example, riding a bike can irritate the perineum and testicles and cause inflammation. Tight sports uniforms can put pressure on the testicles and may cause prostatitis and impotence.[7]

Because of male hormones, men are more prone to develop arteriosclerosis earlier than women. Regular physical exercise can help to slow down the hardening of arteries and can increase the heart's tolerance to physical exercise and labor, which may help prevent heart disease.

Particularly in Western culture, big muscles are perceived as being a sign of masculinity or strength. But, in reality, pushing oneself to consistently lift heavier weights and develop enlarged muscles (which is sometimes accompanied by the use of male hormones, like testosterone) can cause major health problems, such as body pain and heart attack. Enlarged muscles created extra bodyweight that burdens the joints and heart.

Age Appropriate Exercise

Our physical condition and health constantly changes as we age. This has an effect on our bodies' tolerance to different types of physical exercise. Different exercises provide different benefits to the body, depending on our age and the state of our health. Therefore, it is important to develop an age appropriate exercise routine.

Toddlers and young children (one to five years old) –during this time of life children are active, restless and energetic. From the moment they wake-up they are full of energy; because of this, many parents do not think children need structured physical exercise in addition to their normal play. Proper exercise training, however, can effectively train a child to develop lifelong healthy habits and improve their ability to pay attention and get along with others. Some activities for young children may include dance class, swimming lessons, organized youth non-competitive group sports or adult-supervised, structured play dates. Improving a child's ability to concentrate and follow rules in a structured environment is helpful for children with ADD or ADHD.[8] These life skills are not cultivated when children merely partake in unstructured play, especially if they are playing without adult supervision or coaching. This training has the capacity to make a child smarter and more mature because exercise increases the brain's ability to learn new information[9] and participating in group sports helps to develop personal responsibility. It is well known that our personality and character are developed throughout these impressionable young years. Physical activity can influence the route of any child during these transformative years. Additionally, child obesity can start during this age, but if children grow up participating in physical activities, the likelihood of them developing obesity will be greatly reduced because regular exercise will be an important part of their daily lifestyle.

Children and early adolescence (six to fourteen years old) – throughout these years children learn how to pay attention and are eager to learn. Most hobbies and interests are developed during this age. It is good for a child to learn at least two or three different physical sports as hobbies. This is important for the child's health and can influence the rest of their lives. Emotionally, learning to play sports cultivates self-discipline and can increase the child's ability to manage and tolerate stress; a skill that will be useful to them while they are young and as adults. Participating in group sports, such as basketball, soccer, volleyball, football, etc. teaches children social skills and keeps them busy, which means they have less of a chance of developing bad habits as their teammates and coaches may help them cultivate healthy habits such as avoiding drugs and alcohol, eating a healthy diet and keeping up good grades.

It is important to remember to use caution and always put safety first. Sports played during this age must be age-appropriate and the proper protective gear must always be worn. Adequate hydration and other physical protections must be provided with expertise as young children are depending on adults to take care of their needs appropriately. Children should be protected from environmental and weather elements and coaches must be chosen carefully to protect the safety of the children placed in their care. Playing sports, especially group competitive sports, is the best treatment for ADHD. Overall, playing sports from a young age provides a strong foundation for a lifetime of healthy living.

Adolescence to young adulthood (fifteen to twenty-five years old)
–by this age you should already have developed a sports hobby. You
should be healthy and full of energy. Your body should be in peak
physical condition and you should be able to enjoy all kinds of
competitive sports, such as basketball, soccer, volleyball, football,
baseball, karate, etc. This is the age that we find ourselves struggling to
be independent and are busy learning skills or training for a career. Our
life may be unsettled and we may feel that we are under a lot of stress.
Playing sports, especially group sports, can help us relieve life stress,
maintain health, abstain from bad habits, make friends and develop
good social skills. However, because of youthful ambition and lack of
experience, it is common at this age to push your physical limits too far
while playing sports. Sometimes coaches, concerned with competition,
may push young athletes too far or not provide them with the physical
and emotional protection they need. This, unfortunately, may be why
most sports injuries responsible for disability or death happen at this
age. Sports must be played with extra caution. Extreme or dangerous
sports, such as parachute jumping, high ski jumping, rock climbing, dirt
biking, motorcycle jumping, motorcycle racing, etc. should be avoided.
Be smart, don't be a daredevil. No sports thrill is worth jeopardizing
your health or your life.[10]

Adulthood (twenty-five to forty years old) –your physical condition
and tolerance to physical activity gradually begins to decline usually
around this time. Body parts wear and tear easier; therefore, by this age,
you should cut down on extreme competitive physical activity. After
age thirty-five, you should stop playing extreme sports regularly and
should choose different group sports or physical exercise based on
your individual health condition. Unfortunately, most people have a
chronic sports injury by the time they are in their 30's, but with a little
precaution this lifetime pain can be avoided.

Middle-aged adults (forty to sixty-five years old) –during this time
it is common to begin to develop serious arteriosclerosis. Regular,
proper physical activity is one of the best ways to slowdown the
hardening of your arteries. Since your body's tolerance to physical
activity is reduced by this age, you should completely stop playing

extreme competitive sports. Most people already have body pain or injury by this age. Based on your own health condition you can play any or a combination of low-impact sports such as tennis, table tennis, golf, swimming, walking, jogging, snow skiing, hiking, biking, stationary biking, aerobics, water aerobics, tai chi, yoga, etc.

Older adults (over sixty-five years old) –most people will have developed some health problems by the time they are sixty-five years old. Again, it is important to choose an exercise that is appropriate for your health or an exercise program that can be used to treat your health problems. Balance begins to deteriorate during this age, bones are more fragile and the body reacts slower. All of these factors cause us to be more prone to injury at this age. It will take longer to heal when you get injured at this age. Because of this, it is advisable to avoid extreme or competitive sports and sports that require good balance such as ice skating, biking, snow skiing, snowboarding, etc.

Best Physical Activities for Older Adults

Walking is the best exercise for elderly people because it exercises all muscles and joints in the body and is a safe, easy way to maintain balance. Every step you take requires you to balance yourself, which can effectively slow down the deterioration of your balance. Since you are most likely retired by this age, you should be able to walk a few times each day. It is best to walk ten to thirty minutes multiple times throughout the day, as opposed to walking once during the day for an hour or more. Walking more frequently, but for shorter times will help prevent foot and knee injuries. If you have chronic or acute pain in your hips, knees, ankles or feet walking may worsen your pain. Therefore, you should reduce walking or choose another physical activity. If your balance is poor, you should use a cane or a walker to walk. Being careful is better than being sorry. Over 235,000 people fall and fracture their hip each year. Some of these people develop a concussion or fracture their spinal vertebra, pelvis, hand, wrist, arm, ankle or leg as well. Over 500,000 senior citizens require hospitalization after falling each year and hundreds of thousands die directly because of a fall or hip fracture.[11] Clearly, bone fractures can have a serious effect on the health and lives of elderly people.

Stationary bicycles are steady and generally safe for older people to use for exercise. One drawback to using a regular stationary bike is that it doesn't provide upper body exercise. But it does exercise leg muscles and is a good cardiovascular workout. This exercise is appropriate for people who have chronic pain in their legs because stationary cycling reduces stress on the legs caused by carrying bodyweight. Also, it can reduce or prevent edema of the calves and feet. However, people who have prostate problems, urinary tract disorders or hemorrhoids should be cautious when riding a stationary bike because it may irritate or worsen these problems.

A combination of playing golf, tennis, table tennis, light weightlifting, low-impact aerobics, water aerobics, swimming, yoga, tai chi and other similar activities can effectively slow the aging process, keep your mind sharp, maintain good balance, and help keep your muscles and bones strong.

Exercise and Your Career

Too much physical labor or exercise causes damage by wearing down body tissue. You should be conscious of how your work environment, which is where most of us spend the majority of our day, determines which parts of your body you use the most. This information can help you avoid doing the same repetitive motions when you are not working, thus avoiding internal impairment caused by overstraining. The following information can help you develop an exercise routine that can complement the physical demands of your career.

Some professions require hands and fingers to do a lot of repetitive motions, such as working in a nursery, bakery, auto repair, factory or assembly lines; or being a hairdresser, musician, cook, computer programmer or tailor. Some hobbies and exercises also require the use of your hands and fingers, such as riding a motorcycle, playing tennis or racquetball, gardening, knitting, sewing, hand crafts, playing an instrument or hand crafting wood. If your career requires that you use your hands a lot, then you should avoid doing exercises and hobbies that require you to use your hands and fingers too much. This can prevent trigger finger, carpal tunnel syndrome and arthritis in your hands and fingers and more. Activities such as swimming, walking, jogging, hiking, aerobics and water aerobics are more suitable forms of exercise for those who must use their hands in the workplace.

Careers that require a lot of standing or walking, such as cashiers, supply stockers, retail sales, postal or delivery services, security guards, etc. can wear out your hips, knees and feet. After work, these body parts need time to recover and rest so you should avoid walking, jogging, hiking, biking, playing basketball, soccer or football. Activities such as weightlifting, swimming or yoga are better choices for your health.

People who work in construction, farming or other heavy duty physical labor perform enough physical activity while they are working; and therefore, should avoid or reduce extreme physical exercise so as to avoid the chance of internal impairment (wear and tear) caused by overuse. A twenty minute relaxing walk can effectively relieve fatigue and alleviate stress that results from physical labor. Casual walking is perhaps the best choice of exercise for those who spend all day engaged in heavy physical labor.

For careers that demand little to no activity, such as office workers and truck drivers, blood circulation is weakened. In order for your heart to be able to pump blood into your arties and supply your body with the oxygen and nutrients it needs, your muscles need to contract. This contraction of your muscles helps squeeze your blood in your veins back to your heart. When you sit for too long your muscles are less able to effectively circulate your blood. This lack of movement may cause blood stasis in the lower half of your body (pelvic region, legs and feet). Blood stagnation can lead to many different health problems including irregular or painful menstruation, fibroids in the uterus, colitis, constipation, colon ulcers, enlarged prostate, hemorrhoids, foot or hand neuropathy, restless leg syndrome, blood clots in your legs, foot or leg edema, etc. Physical exercise can effectively prevent or treat these health problems and can help relieve stress from work as well as increase you energy and improve efficiency at work. Moderately intense sports are recommended for those who have a more stationary profession, such as walking, jogging, hiking, aerobics, swimming, weightlifting, playing basketball, soccer, tennis, golf, etc. Rotating among these sports is important for your health. Motorcycling, car racing and snowmobiling are less beneficial for those who have stationary jobs.

Exercise and Your Diet

Regular physical exercise can help your digestive system by strengthening the smooth muscles in the intestine and maintaining gastrointestinal peristalsis (the motion made by your intestines to complete the digestion process and move waste out of your body). Regular exercise reduces food intolerances and prevents or reduces arteriosclerosis in your digestive arteries, which is the main cause of indigestion, constipation and nutritional deficiency in elderly people. Exercise affects the health of your digestive system, and, inversely, your diet can determine how exercise will benefit your health. The following are some important points to remember when it comes to diet and its effect on physical exercise.

Avoid doing strenuous exercise after a full meal –physical exercise can stimulate gastrointestinal peristalsis, so strenuous exercise or physical labor performed after a full meal may cause gaging, acid reflux, cramps in the stomach or even a hiatal hernia. If you frequently do strenuous exercise after a full meal you can develop gastritis, indigestion, IBS (Irritable Bowel Syndrome) or acid reflux. You should wait at least one or two hours to do strenuous exercise after eating a full meal.

Avoid strenuous exercise when you are hungry –blood glucose levels are low when you are hungry, so doing strenuous exercise on an empty stomach can cause blood pressure to rapidly rise. It may also lead to fatigue, heart palpitations, increased sweating, dizziness and headaches. Exercising on an empty stomach can also affect you emotionally by reducing your motivation to exercise and making your exercise less enjoyable.

Adjust your caloric intake according to your activity level – because physical exercise burns calories, the more physical exercise or labor you do, the higher your caloric intake should be. The more physical activity you do, the less you have to worry about weight gain and obesity. If you do enough daily physical exercise or labor, you will be able to eat without having to count calories.

Drink plenty of water –you should drink water before, during and after exercise because increased sweating and breathing during physical activities causes more water to be used by your body. Do not wait to drink until you feel thirsty because by the time you feel thirsty you are already dehydrated. It is important to drink water during exercise because it cools your body down and prevents your body from becoming overheated during exercise. Water aids in detoxifying your body, which produces more waste during exercise.

During strenuous exercise you should drink water consistently. However, never drink large amounts to the point where you feel full, because a full stomach may cause you to get stomach cramps. Never drink large amounts of water, especially if you feel extremely thirsty during or after exercise. Drinking too much water can cause your brain to swell and in some cases can even cause death. (See Chapter Two.)

Drinking too much water combined with sweating too much can cause a drop in sodium levels which can be dangerous. If you lose too much of this mineral you will feel fatigued more easily and may even get muscle cramps. If you constantly sweat throughout your exercise routine, especially in hot weather, you should make sure to add a small amount of table salt to your water because you lose sodium and potassium when you sweat, or you can drink a sports drink that has been enhanced to replace these vital nutrients. Some sports drinks are designed to replace the appropriate amount of trace minerals during exercise. It is best to avoid sports drinks that contain artificial colors or other non-essential additives. Don't overuse or misuse sports drinks by thinking of them as "health drinks" appropriate to drink at any time.

You should not drink water that is too purified (lacking minerals) while playing sports. If you sweat a lot, spring or mineral water is better for you than purified water. Do not drink soda to replace water during exercise. Soda can contribute to dehydration and increase thirst. The sugar and citric acid found in soda can irritate your stomach and cause stomach discomfort or acid reflux.

Avoid drinking alcohol –you should avoid drinking alcohol before or during exercise because alcohol can be detrimental to your balance and alertness. It may increase your chance of getting an injury or having an accident during exercise. Your blood pressure and heart rate rise during exercise, which means alcohol can cause more damage to your arteries and your heart. Drinking alcohol may force your liver to work harder as well.

Exercise and Seasonal Changes

Weather can affect blood circulation and breathing as well as affect the results of exercise. Making adjustments and taking precautions based on weather conditions should allow you to participate in a healthy and rewarding exercise program year-round.

Winter

Cold weather can inconvenience your outdoor exercise and can greatly affect your health. Cold weather can slow down your blood circulation. Reduced blood circulation means slower oxygen and nutrition supply, and slower detoxification of your body. Cold temperatures can lower your body's tolerance to physical exercise, increase stiffness, pain or inflammation in your joints. If you already have joint pain or body aches you should avoid doing exercise in cold weather. However, you can comfortably exercise in cold weather by dressing adequately and staying warm during outdoor exercise. Make sure to wear extra layers over any painful joints you may have. Tolerance to physical activity is lowered in cold temperatures, so in order to avoid injuries during cold weather you should avoid playing extreme sports such as basketball, soccer, football, volleyball, baseball, etc.

The ground may be icy or slippery when the temperature is below freezing. This can increase your risk of slipping or falling. Older people in particular should avoid or reduce outdoor activity during wintertime because their balance is poor and their bones are fragile. Young people can more easily enjoy winter sports, such as skiing, snowshoeing, ice skating, ice hockey, etc.

Winter sports are fun, but can also be dangerous and risky. Skiing, ski jumping and snowboarding can result in severe injuries such as bone fracture, paralysis and even death.[12] You must be properly trained by a professional so that if you choose to ski or snowboard, you may do so safely. Snowmobiling has barely any health benefits, but has many risks for injury such as rolling over, getting lost or stuck, getting caught in an avalanche, falling, losing control or excessive speed leading to an impact, etc. All of these types of snowmobiling accidents happen in the United States annually.[13]

Pollution, fog and inversions are worse in winter, especially in big cities. You should avoid or reduce outdoor exercise when the air quality is bad. Cold air can irritate the respiratory system, which can cause a runny nose, stuffy nose, cough and asthma attacks. Because cold air has to be warmed up before it enters your lungs, it can irritate or "freeze" your upper respiratory organs such as your nasal cavities, pharynx and wind pipe causing inflammation or an allergic reaction in your respiratory system, especially if you breathe in too deeply and too quickly during strenuous exercise. Wearing a warm and thick mask can help you warm the air and protect your nose from frostbite. Avoid or reduce doing strenuous exercise in freezing weather, especially if you already have a respiratory disorder, because your respiratory system's tolerance to cold weather will be lower than normal.

Due to reduced blood circulation your blood vessels are more rigid and tense causing your blood pressure to rise during cold weather. That is why the rate of heart attack is highest during winter months. If you have high blood pressure, are at a high risk for having a heart attack or you already have heart problems, you should use extra caution when exercising outdoors and avoid doing strenuous exercise in cold weather.

Summer

Temperatures are high during summer. If you do not properly plan your physical exercise for hot weather, you can damage your health. Your body produces heat during exercise, especially during strenuous exercise. When the temperature is high, as it is during summer, it is more difficult to cool down. The body cools itself down quickly by sweating. This is why it is important to drink enough water during outdoor physical exercise in warm weather. When the temperature is extremely hot (more than 90 degrees Fahrenheit), you should reduce or avoid doing outdoor exercise because your body's tolerance to physical exercise will be reduced. This is especially true for older people because the body's ability to adjust to heat decreases with age. Heat can cause fatigue, body ache, heat exhaustion and heat stroke.

A mild sun bath is good for your health. It can promote your body to make vitamin D and is good for emotional health, but too much sunshine can damage your skin by speeding up the aging process, increasing wrinkles and causing skin cancer. Too much sun exposure can cause eye damage such as macular degeneration or cataracts, which cause vision loss. The sun's rays are stronger in summer and contain high levels of radiation (ultraviolet light). So you should prepare accordingly before going outdoors. Make sure to wear ultraviolet protection sunglasses, a loose and long sleeve UV blocking shirt, long, loose pants and a brimmed sun blocking hat. When you go swimming outdoors you should put sunscreen on all areas of your skin that will be exposed to sunshine. Many people make the mistake that on cloudy days it is safe to be without sun block protection, but clouds only partially block ultraviolet rays. You should protect yourself well even in cloudy weather.

Prevent yourself from getting bitten by insects and small animals during outdoor exercise. Insect bites can cause serious health problems, like allergic reactions, skin irritation and some types of long-term diseases such as West Nile Virus or Lyme disease. When you go outdoors in wooded areas, such as in the mountains, you should wear long pants to protect yourself from plant scratches and insects. Make sure to check your clothes for ticks during or after hiking. In order to avoid mosquito bites you should wear protective clothing (long-sleeved shirt and pants), avoid outdoor exercise after sunset and avoid getting too close to plants or crops where insects usually feed.

Avoid swimming in polluted or infested rivers or lakes, especially in areas with warmer climates or in developing countries so as to avoid coming into contact with pollution, bacteria, parasites or viruses.

Because it is hot during summer, some people enjoy cooling off after physical exercise, but being too cold can negatively affect your health. The water in a river or lake can be very cold. Swimming in cold water can cause body aches or pains, joint stiffness and afterwards can cause you to get a fever or develop a cold. It is true that drinking cold water can cool down your body temperature during or after physical exercise, but drinking warm or room temperature water is healthier. Cold water, especially ice-cold water, can cause heartburn, digestive system irritation, gastritis or cramps in your stomach. Avoid taking a cold shower after exercise, especially when you are sweating and still hot from exercise. Taking a cold shower when you are still hot from exercise may cause body aches or discomfort. Make sure to change your clothes if they are wet from sweat, rain or water. A drop in your body temperature caused by wet clothing can cause muscle aches or discomfort later. If you go fly fishing make sure to wear the right type of warm and waterproof pants or else the cold water may cause foot or leg pain and cramping. Standing in cold water too often can cause osteoarthritis and fibromyalgia.

Rain, wind, thunder and lightning storms occur more frequently in summer. Outdoor exercises should be avoided during extreme weather conditions. Wind can stir up dust, pollen and pollution in the air. Cold rain on your head and body can cause headaches, body aches and cold syndrome. Avoid exercising outdoors during a wind storm because wind stirs up dust that can get into and irritate your eyes and respiratory system. Irritation or inflammation in your respiratory system can trigger allergic reactions. Also, wind can break tree branches and blow down trees which can cause serious injuries.

Spring

Temperatures change frequently during spring. This makes it difficult to dress appropriately for exercising outside. Many people catch colds during spring because they do not wear clothing that is warm enough. You should always check the outside temperature before going to exercise outdoors and make sure to dress warm enough or carry a jacket with you.

Pollen levels are high in spring. Many people are sensitive or allergic to these substances so you should avoid or reduce outdoor exercise if you notice that you are sensitive to pollen. To reduce allergy syndrome you can exercise indoors, use an air purifier in your exercise room and use warm water to rinse your eyes and nose after exercise.

If you are inactive during winter your muscles and heart will not be ready for strenuous exercise in spring. You should gradually increase your physical exercise before doing strenuous activity to avoid muscle pain or injury.

Autumn

As the temperature gradually decreases during autumn make sure to dress accordingly when you exercise outdoors during this season. It is more likely that you will catch a cold if you do not wear warm enough clothing. Although the temperature is cooling, sunshine is still strong so make sure to wear good sunglasses, protective gear and clothing that protect your eyes and skin from sun exposure.

Scheduling Your Exercise Program

If you make exercise a regular part of your schedule, exercise will more easily become part of you lifelong habit and make it easier for your body to accept and perform exercise. For example, exercise can be more enjoyable and easier to stick to if you exercise regularly with a friend or family member. If you are randomly and infrequently invited by your friends to exercise, it will most likely be less pleasant, more tiring and physically more difficult for your body to perform. The following are suggestions for scheduling your exercise routine based on time of day.

Early morning –is a good time to do low-impact, physical exercise, such as walking, stationary biking, stretching exercises or light weightlifting. You should make sure to drink some water before you exercise because you can get dehydrated in the morning after not drinking for many hours during sleep. A session of twenty to thirty minutes of exercise should be good enough. Avoid strenuous exercise in the morning, especially extreme competitive sports, because your body is dehydrated and requires more nutrition and your brain and body need more time to wake up, so your attention and ability to react may be low. Strenuous exercise can be very difficult for your body to perform in the early morning and you may feel more fatigued throughout the rest of the day after doing strenuous exercise in the morning. Your body's blood circulation is reduced during sleep, but warm-up exercises can promote blood circulation and detoxify your body in the morning. The right kind of gently, warming exercises can help you feel better and more energized throughout the rest of the day.

Noon to late afternoon –is the warmest time of day in winter or cold weather regions. Sunshine is the strongest during this time so you should wear sunscreen and sun blocking clothes. During summer you should avoid or reduce outdoor physical exercise between noon and about 4 p.m. because the sun's rays are most intense during this time of day.

Evening –is the best time of day to exercise, especially if you are performing strenuous exercise or extreme competitive sports, because the oxygen level in the air is highest in the evening. Plus, exercise can burn all the extra calories that you did not use during the day. The fatigue caused by exercise can help you sleep better at night. But you should avoid doing strenuous exercise one hour before going to bed because your body needs time to cool down and relax before sleeping.

You should not lie down when you are sweating from exercise because it can cause blood stasis in your body and lead to discomfort or pain.

Choosing the Right Exercise Clothing

Exercise clothes should be loose and comfortable. Wearing clothes that are too tight can cause pressure and squeeze or irritate body tissue causing discomfort, fatigue and inflammation. Wearing a tight head band, tight eyeglass frames or cords can cause headache. Wearing a sports bra that is too tight can cause neck, shoulder and upper back pain. Wearing an elastic belt around the waist line that is too tight can cause lower back pain. Wearing a knee brace that is too tight can cause fatigue or discomfort in your calves. Clothes that are too tight can also affect your flexibility while playing sports.

Wear season appropriate exercise clothing. For example, you should dress warmly to exercise outdoors because exposure to cold can stiffen your joints, lower your body's physical tolerance and may increase your risk of getting hurt. In summer, you should wear sun blocking clothing. In spring and fall, because of the rapid temperature change, you should layer your clothing and be prepared for rapid weather changes.

Exercise clothing should be loose and have good air flow. Your muscles produce a lot of body heat during exercise. Good air flow in between your skin and clothing can help you cool down easier and faster. The material exercise clothing is made out of should absorb sweat easily such as cotton. Some materials that do not absorb sweat will stick and rub against your skin, which can be very distracting. Your exercise clothing should fit you, but not too tightly.

Change sweat soaked clothes as soon as possible after you are finished exercising. Wearing wet clothes can increase muscle fatigue and discomfort.

Wearing the appropriate shoes for the activity you are participating in is absolutely necessary for comfortable and effective exercise. Exercise shoes should not be too tight or too small for your feet. Tight shoes squeeze your feet and affect the blood circulation in your feet causing pain, potentially ingrown toenails, damaged toe nails and hammer toes. If your shoes are too loose while you exercise your feet will slide forwards and backwards causing scratching, irritation and blisters. Also, the chance of tripping and losing your balance is more likely. The soles of your shoes should be spongy, elastic and cushiony and should provide good support for your feet, especially if you exercise on concrete or wood floors. Hard soles can cause neuroma and plantar fasciitis. You should also make sure that the bottoms of your exercise shoes have adequate traction, especially if you exercise on a smooth wood floor or frozen ground because you may slip or fall. The heel of exercise shoes should not be too high; the higher the heel, the higher the chance will be for you to sprain your ankle.

Make sure to wear the appropriate protective gear. Wear a helmet and protective clothing when you play certain extreme sports, such as football, baseball, hockey, biking, motorcycling, boxing, etc. Always make sure children you responsible for are properly fitted with protective gear suitable for the sport they are playing as well.

Choosing the Best Exercise Environment

The environment that you exercise in is very important. You must make sure to exercise in surroundings that provide fresh air, a sense of relaxation and safety. How can you determine whether or not the air is fresh? You can use your nose, eyes and brain to make sure you exercise in the best possible air quality available to you.

1. Do not exercise near traffic or busy roads. Car exhaust contains all kinds of potentially toxic and carcinogenic gases;[14] inhaling polluted air is bad for your health.

2. Fertilizer, pesticides, paint and other household chemicals, especially ones that are sprayed, can pollute the air. If you see or smell these pollutants you should avoid exercising in these environments.

3. Flower pollen and various other plants put pollutants into the air. Many people are allergic to pollen. But even if you are not allergic to pollen, inhaling these substances can still be bad for your health.

4. Overall, outdoor air is fresher than indoor air due to the use of cleaning products, accumulation of dust and dirt in and around furniture and outgassing from household items such as plastics and furniture.

5. Do not exercise in foggy or windy weather conditions or during inversions.

6. Do not exercise outdoors when air quality is poor or if smoke is present from forest fires, wood burnings stoves, etc.

7. Use extra caution if you play sports that require the use of a gas motor (such as snowmobiling, watercraft, car racing, etc.). These vehicles produce pollution. The waste (exhaust) created by these vehicles may damage your health if inhaled. For example, a man I know took his son and friend water skiing. His son was sitting by the motor and passed out. After they rushed the boy to the hospital, the doctor informed the father that the reason the boy fainted was that the boy breathed in too much exhaust from the boat's motor.

8. Chlorine used in public swimming pools can irritate your respiratory system and your skin. Chlorine may even cause long-term respiratory and skin health problems for some people.[15]

9. Bars and dance clubs are usually filled with fragrant odors from people's perfumes and cigarette smoke; these establishments are usually not a good place to do a lot of physical exercise (dancing). Oxygen levels may be reduced in these enclosed spaces because they are usually densely crowded and poorly ventilated.

You should use your cognitive skills to determine whether or not the air you breathe is suitable for exercise activities. The less fragrant and foreign substances there are in the air, the less chemicals you will ingest and the better the air is for your health.

Exercise in a Safe Environment

1. Do not ride a bike, rollerblade, skateboard or run on the side of a busy road. If you crash or trip and fall in the line of traffic you can be seriously injured. Even if you stay in the pedestrian lanes there are many careless, distracted, drowsy or drunk drivers on the road that may cross over the line and hit you.

2. Do not play sports on uneven ground. The chance of spraining your ankle is higher when you run on uneven ground.

3. Whitewater rafting, rock climbing, steep cliff jumping, parachute jumping, skiing or snowmobiling in unknown areas and dirt biking on steep hills are all sports that take place in dangerous environments. These activities should be avoided in order to preserve your health and safety.

4. How can you find a relaxing environment appropriate for exercise? First, make sure that you have cultivated an environment that allows you to place all your attention and focus on your activity. Do not watch TV, listen to music, talk or sing while you exercise. These activities lessen your focus during exercise. Do not exercise around noisy machines or traffic. Avoid playing sports with somebody who has a negative attitude (grumpy, bad tempered, violent or mean spirited). Negative emotions can seriously affect how beneficial your exercise can be for you.

Prepare for Exercise

1. Be well prepared for outdoor exercise. Wear proper clothing and always carry drinking water. For wilderness activities bring snacks, a raincoat and other essential items and wear appropriate closed-toe tennis shoes or hiking boots.

2. Do not exercise when you are too hungry or too full. Remember, you should not do strenuous exercise an hour before or after a meal.

3. Do a warm-up exercise before extreme, competitive exercise. Warm-up exercises gradually increase the blood circulation in your body and prepare your body for extreme physical exercise. This helps reduces the risk of having a rapid rise in your blood pressure that can cause headaches, vision damage, heart attack or shock. Warm-up exercises can loosen up your muscles and joints and help you avoid injury. Taking a slow run, a fast-paced walk or stretching for five to ten minutes are all good ways to warm-up.

4. Be consistent, plan and make exercise a regular activity. Make an appointment with yourself to exercise and keep it faithfully. Once you have a routine, exercise simply becomes a part of your internal clock and your body can handle it much better.

5. You should be aware of your body's individual tolerance to physical exercise. If you are not active or you do not exercise regularly you should be cautious when you begin to exercise so as to avoid body aches and pain. For example, if you are not trained to run an eight hundred meter race but you just go and run the race, the sudden increase in activity can cause your blood pressure to rise rapidly, give you a headache, and can even cause you to go into shock. This sudden increase in activity can cause you to develop disinsertion (sudden blindness) or have a heart attack. If you train for a month before the race your body will be able to handle the race much better. For elderly people in particular, exercise or extreme exercise can trigger a heart attack.

After Participating in Sports or Exercise

1. Cool down after exercise. As you play extreme sports you breathe harder and your heart beats faster because your cells require more rapid blood circulation in order to supply more oxygen and nutrients to your muscles and quickly secrete metabolic waste. After you stop playing, your body needs a little time to cool down and recover so your body tissue cells can continue to clean themselves and excrete waste. Walking for ten minutes is the best way to cool down after exercise and can prevent body fatigue and body aches.

2. Do not sit down right after exercise, especially after playing extreme competitive sports, because it may increase your chance of bursitis in your buttocks or sciatica (pinched nerve that causes leg pain). From my experience working with dozens of competitive runners, sitting after exercise is a common cause of sciatica.

3. Do not take a cold shower right after exercise. It can cause you to have body aches or develop a cold. Avoid taking too hot of a bath right after exercise because it can increase body fatigue or muscle aches later. It is best to take a lukewarm shower or bath after strenuous exercise. (Magnesium sulfate commonly known as Epsom salts added to your bath may help reduce muscle pain as well.)

4. If you sweat a lot make sure to change your clothes right after you exercise. Wet clothes can cause body aches and cold syndrome to emerge later.

5. You should dress and keep warm after exercise so that your body maintains good blood circulation. This will help your body recover from having physically exerted itself.

6. Your body needs time to recover from the physical injury of exercise. Resting well is the best thing you can do to help your body recover from physical injury. If you exercise again or engage in physical labor soon after exercise your chance of having a repetitive injury will be higher because you are not giving your body enough time to recover. As is well known, you should listen to your body, and be aware of your body's tolerance to physical injury.

7. Avoid exercising, especially extreme competitive sports, after performing hard labor. Too much physical activity can make you feel tired, so allow yourself time to rebuild your energy before you begin playing sports or exercising again.

8. Remember not to drink a large amount of ice-cold water immediately after playing sports or exercising. Cold water may help you cool down faster, but cold water can cause your stomach muscles to spasm. This damage can take a few days to recover from, so it is best to drink warm or room temperature water after strenuous physical activities.

How Individual Types of Exercise Affect Your Health

Walking is one of the best exercises and it is suitable for most people. Walking exercises nearly every muscle in your body, effectively detoxifies your body, promotes good energy and is incredibly safe. Perhaps walking causes the least amount of physical injury because our bodies are designed to walk. Walking is appropriate for people of all ages and is the best exercise to maintain balance for seniors. However, no sport is perfect. Walking too much can cause foot neuroma (foot pain), plantar fasciitis (heel pain) and joint damage.

My recommendation for people who are over sixty-five years old, overweight or obese, pregnant (over five months), or have rheumatoid arthritis, lupus, foot pain, knee pain or hip pain is to be extra cautious before starting a walking program. Avoid walking long distances or for extended periods of time. If you have a daily exercise time goal, it is better to plan to take several short walks throughout the day instead of taking one long walk. For example, it will be easier your body to tolerate taking a twenty minute walk in the morning, afternoon and evening instead of walking one hour all at once. Remember to pay attention to how your body feels and make decisions based on what will be most beneficial for your health.

Stationary bicycling is a good cardiovascular exercise. It helps your body to detoxify and maintain energy. It is performed indoors, which means weather and outdoor temperature changes cannot interfere with your exercise routine. It is safe and there is no need to worry about falling. Stationary bicycling takes the weight off your lower body and corresponding joints, so it is a good way to relieve physical stress from your legs and feet. Stationary biking exercise requires you to pump your calves and feet encouraging increased circulation. This effectively helps pump blood back to your heart and can prevent and treat calf and foot edema. Older people who have swelling of the feet can treat this by exercising on a stationary bike for five to ten minutes once every hour or every other hour. Since stationary bicycling does not exercise the upper body, you can add light weights to your routine to build your upper body strength. If you have a urinary tract disorder, hemorrhoids or prostate problems you should be extra careful while biking because the bike seat may irritate your genital area and worsen these problems.

Outdoor bicycling can be a positive social activity because you can invite friends or family to enjoy a bike ride with you. Pedal bikes are an environmentally friendly form of transportation. In fact, in some countries bicycles are still used as the main mode of transportation. Biking is a sport that requires balance. Regardless of how skilled you are at riding, you still run the risk of falling for various unexpected reasons. Because of this, seniors and those who have osteoporosis should not ride bicycles. Weather conditions can make biking more dangerous. Windy weather makes it more difficult to ride and increases the chances of falling. Rain can hinder vision and make the road slippery. Choose good weather conditions before you go out for a bike ride. Biking can be dangerous; if you fall you can fracture or break a bone. Biking places stress and tension on your hands and neck may lead to trigger finger, carpal tunnel syndrome, wrist pain and neck pain. Bicycling may worsen pain for those who have a knee injury. Make sure you wear a helmet to protect your head and avoid jumping or risky riding. When mountain biking, wear clothing that can effectively protect you from bush scratches, rubbing up against various plants, bug bites and skin injuries caused by falling.

Running or Jogging provide health benefits similar to walking. Running is a good cardiovascular exercise because it increases your heart's tolerance to physical activity; therefore strengthening it and reducing your resting heart rate. Running strengthens your lungs' air capacity & ability to exchange oxygen (breathe), balances your immune system and effectively treats and prevents autoimmune disorders such as asthma. Running can help balance your appetite. For those who have a poor appetite, running can increase it. For those who have too active of an appetite, running can reduce it. Running balances your endorphin levels. This can reduce stress or pain and helps balance emotional disorders such as depression, anxiety, anger, etc. and can balance hormonal thyroid problems. However, like every activity, you have to run moderately or else it can damage your health. While running all of your bodyweight comes down on your hips, knees, ankles and feet. This pounding pressure can amount to several times your bodyweight. Repeated pounding pressure on your joints can increase the rate of wear and tear of your body.

Avoid or reduce running if you have hip, knee, ankle or foot problems. Be moderate with how long you run if you are overweight. Running twenty minutes a day, but no longer than two hours total per week is fine for a young and healthy person.

If you take up running, you must allow your body muscles and heart to slowly build up tolerance. A healthy person who begins running might experience shortness of breath, fatigue, no enjoyment and soreness the next day for the first month. But, if you keep it up, you will slowly become accustomed to running and your body will adjust to it. If you have uncontrolled high blood pressure you should not run. Running raises your blood pressure which may increase your risk of having a stroke or heart attack.

Running too much can damage your heart. One of my patients asked me whether or not it is it healthy to run a marathon. I explained to her that the first man who ran what is now the distance of a marathon died right after he completed the feat.[16] In my opinion, running a marathon is not good for your overall heart health. You should try to avoid running more than thirty minutes at one time.

Since running balances endorphin levels, it can be a very addictive form of exercise. It may take a while to begin to enjoy running, but later it can be very difficult to quit or abstain from it. You must use your willpower to control yourself and run for only a healthy amount of time. If running becomes more of a health problem than a benefit, you should reduce how much you run or quit running altogether. Too much running can cause an imbalance in your hormones, for women this can cause irregular menstruation and can decrease infertility.

Playing basketball has the same health benefits as running, plus additional health benefits. Basketball teaches self-discipline because there are many rules to follow. This makes it a good sport for preteens and teenagers who may have personal or social issues or conflicts. The players must learn how to play as a team and get along with each other. Because it is a team sport, it cultivates good social skills and often leads to long-term friendships. Playing on a basketball team can assist in the treatment ADHD because the sport requires full attention and concentration during a game.[17]

During a basketball game players can be under a lot of pressure to win or perform well. Dealing with this pressure regularly during games can help build up tolerance to stress which can be beneficial for life events that occur at school or in the workplace. It is a good, clean and healthy hobby. But, like all other sports, you must play basketball moderately. Remember that a serious injury can cause you to never be able to play again. Don't sacrifice your health for sport. Basketball can cause the same injuries as running, as well as others. Because basketball involves a lot of jumping, twisting, sudden shifts in acceleration and falling, spraining a knee or ankle is very common. It is an extremely competitive and sometimes violent sport, and only younger people should play it.

Once you reach about 40 years of age, you should stop playing competitive basketball. If you have already injured yourself or if you have pain related to playing, you should not participate in a basketball game because your body will favor the opposite side of your injured body part, essentially placing an unbalanced amount of stress on that side, potentially leading to another injury. It is best when you have been injured to rest and not play again until your injury has fully healed. Because basketball can be somewhat violent, you should wear a mouth guard, especially during high school, college or professional basketball games to avoid losing a tooth or getting some other type of mouth injury.

Because of the social elements and higher level of excitement obtained from scoring points, playing basketball can be more enjoyable and more addictive than running. Never intentionally try to hurt other players physically or emotionally. Be aware of how your words and actions affect the other players. Use common sense to protect yourself during the game. If you sense danger, you should avoid the challenge. Remember to play smart. Avoid playing with bullies, people who are rude or violent. They will only bring you stress and tension, which is not good for your health. Make sure to cover any cuts or open wounds with bandages to avoid getting viruses transmitted by sweat. Have a positive attitude while you play basketball. If you do not enjoy playing the sport, then do not play. If you play because you simply cannot stop or for money then you should seriously reconsider your motives.

Playing soccer has pretty much the same health benefits as playing basketball, but it exercises the upper body less. Because of this, there are less shoulder injuries in soccer than in basketball. However, soccer can damage your feet, especially the foot you use to kick the ball. When you kick the ball, there is compressed pressure between the foot and the hard soccer ball. Repeatedly kicking powerfully or serving long-distance can cause damage to your foot. In order to protect your feet, do not play soccer without shoes. It is best to wear soccer shoes during play.

A common injury in soccer is injury to the shinbone, which results from the shin being kicked, bumped or scratched by the sole of another player's shoe. It is imperative that you wear a good pair of protective long socks (or shin guards) to cover your shinbone (also known as the tibia or shankbone).

If you are not familiar with the field you are about to play on, make sure to check it for uneven ground, bumps and holes before you play so that you can decrease your chance of spraining your knee or ankle.

Soccer is mainly an outdoor game. As with all outdoor sporting activities, you should avoid playing soccer in extreme weather conditions including during rain or windy weather, after rain or during extremely cold or hot temperatures. It is best to not play in outdoor areas that are polluted or have poor air quality.

Football has some of the same health benefits as basketball and soccer, but it is definitely a more violent sport. Because football involves impact, there are some things to keep in mind and be cautious of when playing. Wear a helmet to reduce your risk of getting a concussion, which can cause massive brain damage and increase your chances of developing dementia later in life.[18] Do not play when you are fatigued or drowsy. When you are tired your response time is slowed and, therefore, you have an increased chance of being injured. Football is played mainly outdoors; like other outdoor sports, you should make sure to dress appropriately depending on the weather conditions. During cold weather games make sure to warmly dress your joints to prevent them from stiffening. Do not try to gain weight for the game. As I explained earlier, the more weight (whether it is fat or muscle weight) you have, the worse it is for your heart health.

Tennis is both an independent and social sport and because it requires less people in order to be able to play and is much easier to organize and carry out then most other games. Because playing tennis is less violent than other sports, there is less chance that you will injure your body while playing tennis. This is why many people can continue to play tennis well into their 80's. Playing tennis can cause tennis elbow, trigger finger, carpal tunnel syndrome and shoulder pain. Another common injury for tennis players is knee injury.

Winter sports including skiing, snowboarding, ice skating, ice hockey, sledding, snowshoeing and snowmobiling can be good physical workouts and are exciting, joyful sports that make getting through long, cold winters easier. However, there are a few important tips to remember when choosing a winter activity.

Skiing, snowboarding, ice skating and ice hockey require the participant to have good balance. Experiencing a fall while playing these sports is not just a chance, it is a certainty. That is, no matter how good you are, you will fall at some point while playing these sports. About ten out of every one thousand skiers or snowboarders receive an injury that requires immediate medical treatment each year.[19] Ice skating wears out the joints in your legs, which is why professional figure skaters should stop competing by the age of twenty-five. Ice hockey is one of the most violent sports because it involves a lot of hitting, pushing, bumping and shoving; also, it involves a lot of speed skating, stopping and sharp turning, which can cause great physical damage to your body. If you are sixty-five years old or older or if you have osteoporosis, knee or hip problems, you should not play these sports.

Most winter sports are played outdoors. Make sure to dress warmly and actively prevent frostbite and sunburns. Snowmobiling is dangerous. Each year thousands of snowmobiling accidents are caused by crashing into trees, rolling over, sinking or falling into water, getting stuck or lost somewhere, vehicle malfunction or breakdown or by being buried by avalanches. These accidents result in thousands of injuries and over one hundred deaths each year.[20]

Sledding is a fun activity for children, but it can be dangerous if done without supervision. Make sure to pick a safe place with no obstacles such as tress, buildings, parked cars or traffic. Snowshoeing is a good workout and is safe for all ages. Dress warmly and make sure to protect your skin from sun exposure.

Golf is a fairly social sport. It is gentle on your body and doesn't require physical contact with other players, making it appropriate for all ages. However, neck, shoulder, elbow, back and knee injuries can occur if you practice or play too much. If you have any of these problems, reduce how often you play or stop playing altogether. For younger people, golf is probably not the most efficient physical exercise because they often do not have the time required to play golf.

Boxing, kickboxing, karate, gong fu and wrestling are good physical workouts that teach self-defense skills and build self-confidence. These are the most violent sports precisely because the goal is to attack your opponent. Excessively violent fighting can cause brain damage (boxer dementia is well known) and injuries to your kidneys, heart, liver, digestive system, breast glands, testicles, jaw joints, neck, shoulders, wrists, knees, hips, ankles and feet. Playing these sports guarantees that your will be impacted, especially during training. Repetitive motion and pounding can be very hard on your body. Keep in mind that the older you are, the less your body will be able to tolerate. I suggest abstaining from fighting matches after age thirty-five. There are other ways to approach self-defense that can teach you how to avoid unnecessary violence and physical conflict. It is important to educate yourself about low or non-violent self-defense options.

Water sports such as swimming, water aerobics and snorkeling are good physical exercises for those who are overweight or have hip, knee or foot problems. The water alleviates how much weight is put on your lower body. However, swimming too much can cause neck or shoulder injury from the repetitive motion of certain strokes. If you already have neck or shoulder pain, you should reduce how often you swim. Be aware that the chlorine used in public swimming pools can severely irritate your skin and lungs. If you have respiratory disorders or sensitive skin, you should be extra cautious when you swim at public facilities. On the other hand, swimming in salty ocean or lake water can also irritate your skin. Swimming in cold water can stiffen your joints, lower your body's tolerance to physical activity, lower the effectiveness of your immune system and raise your blood pressure. Do not swim in dirty lake or river water in order to avoid getting a bacterial, viral, parasitic or other infection. Because water gets into ear and nasal cavities, swimmers have a higher chance of getting swimmer's ear and nasal infections. If you already have ear, eye, nose or sinus issues you should avoid swimming because the water may contain bleach or germs that can irritate your pre-existing conditions.

Backpacking, rock climbing or mountain and trail hiking are all fun, but strenuous forms of physical exercise. These sports can be best enjoyed if you are in good physical condition, prepared with essential equipment and properly trained before going out.

Hiking is a heart healthy hobby that can help you relax and enjoy nature. But hiking can be hard on your knees as well. If you have knee problems, you should avoid hiking too much. Make sure you choose a safe trail to hike on, avoid steep hillsides and make sure you are not directly above or next to a cliff or river. Muddy, icy, snowy or very sandy, rocky and bumpy trails can increase your chances of tripping or falling. Be aware that you may run into snakes, insects and other animals that may attack you if you accidently startle them. If you are an amateur mountaineer, it is best to stick to popular and maintained trails. Always carry water, extra clothing and other essentials items with you when hiking.

Rock climbing is fun and safe when proper and modern gear is used. Climbing without gear in the wilderness can be very dangerous. Although it is exciting for some people, you should know that fatal accidents happen to rock climbers every year.[21] If you have carpal tunnel syndrome, trigger finger, arthritis in your hands, shoulder or leg pain, you should avoid this sport. If you want to experience rock climbing, you should first be properly trained (perhaps at an indoor facility) and bring an experienced climber with you when you go on your first climb.

Climbing mountains and backpacking can be good cardio workouts and social sports. However, you must be in excellent health and well prepared before you take up mountain climbing. It is best to go with someone who has climbing experience just in case you have mountain sickness, get lost, have an accident, experience an avalanche, etc.

Backpacking is a physically difficult activity and the weight of the backpack can cause back and neck pain.

Moderate weightlifting is a healthy cardio exercise. If done properly, it can strengthen muscles and bones. Performed under professional training, it can effectively treat certain illnesses. For example, strong abdominal muscles can help heal a hernia and strong quadriceps can treat certain types of knee pain. As discussed earlier in this chapter, muscles that are too large can be a burden for your heart and joints. Healthy weightlifting does not aim to make your muscles bigger, but rather aims to make your muscles stronger. Lifting too heavy of a weight can cause injuries such as sprained or torn muscles, shoulder or neck pain and hernias. Again, it is best learn how to weightlift from a professional trainer. Weightlifting for injury treatment should be done under the direct supervision of a medical professional.

Key Points to Remember to Get the Best Health Benefit From Exercise

Choose activities that fit your individual health needs. Different exercises are appropriate for different people. If you do not choose the correct exercise you may end up doing more harm than good to your body. Your exercise plan and schedule should be based on your health, age, career demands and weight.

Your motive to exercise should always be to improve or maintain your health. Do not use exercise solely as a way to gain money, reward and attention or because you are addicted to the way it makes you feel.

Alternate between different types of sports as a way to prevent injuries caused by repetitive motion. For example, running twenty minutes, swimming twenty minutes and spending twenty minutes weightlifting every day is much better than solely running, swimming or weightlifting for one hour at a time.

Choose sports that are safe. Some sports are dangerous, thereby making them unhealthy fitness choices for most people. Car or motorcycle racing, parachute jumping, rock climbing, high ski jumping, snowboarding and other extreme sports cause more injuries and fatalities than less intense activities. No matter how careful you are, you still put yourself in danger when you do these activities. One of my patients who raced motorcycles told me how he saw people, including many of his friends, get broken bones, become paralyzed (some of them becoming paraplegic or quadriplegic) or die because of racing. This patient had one knee fracture and four slipped neck vertebrae from two different motorcycle crashes. He told me, "I was fearless when I started motorcycle racing, now that I am more experienced and see the injuries it can cause, I am more afraid."

Playing sports and exercise are not the same things. Most sports were not created for health purposes and were probably not started by health-wise professionals either. Participate in activities that promote whole-body health. Sports like running marathons, gymnastics, wrestling, boxing, parachute jumping and most extreme competitive sports such as playing basketball, soccer, football, baseball, etc. were developed with fun and enjoyment in mind. It is best for the preservation of your health not to play these sports every day. Instead, choose walking, swimming, low-impact aerobics, tai chi, yoga and other more relaxing, yet effective forms of exercise as part of your daily routine.

Health Benefits of Exercise

Physical exercise is very important for blood circulation. Your body is designed to move. Moving helps your heart pump blood (oxygen and nutrients) throughout your body. Because of gravity, the blood in your veins needs muscles to contract in order to pump blood back to your heart and excrete waste out of your body. If you do not exercise, some parts of your body can develop circulation stasis, in which tissue cells lack oxygen and nutrition and their waste cannot be excreted, thus making these cells sick and unhealthy. This is why people who are not physically active are more tired, feel more pain and get sick more often. In order to stay healthy, you must maintain blood circulation in every part of your body. Walking is the best form of exercise for health maintenance.

Exercise can improve your energy level. Because exercise maintains and improves blood circulation, your body is better able to supply body tissue cells with the oxygen and nutrients they need. This explains why active people feel more energy.

Exercise detoxifies your body. Your body's tissue cells are constantly producing waste (metabolic waste). This waste is toxic to your body. Blood circulation transports this waste to sites where it will then be excreted through bowel movements, urination, exhalation or sweat. Exercising regularly will help keep your body detoxified.

Exercise maintains and strengthens your immune system. Your immune system is your body's defense system. In order to perform its duty, blood needs to transport antibodies, white blood cells and carrier cells to the site of infection. Blood circulation also supplies nutrition to repair injured body tissue. Just like during war, we must be able to transport soldiers, weapons and supplies to the frontline. Without a good transportation system, we can easily lose the war. Exercise can prevent and treat inflammation of autoimmune diseases, which are the result of an inefficient or confused immune system.

Exercise increases the amount of calories you burn and balances your metabolism. Burning more calories can combat and prevent or reverse complications caused by metabolic syndrome such as high blood pressure, high cholesterol, insulin resistance, diabetes and obesity.

Exercise is enjoyable and entertaining. It may also be considered as an effective and pleasing treatment for emotional disorders. Enjoying a sport creates positive emotions, which effectively combat negative emotions such as depression, anger, stress and anxiety because exercise helps to balances endorphin levels. Physical health is the basis of mental health. Often, depression is the result or side-effect of poor physical health. Exercise can reduce stress and anxiety, as well as occupy the mind by leaving less time and energy to think depressing thoughts. Because sports require full attention they are a great way to manage ADHD and other attention disorders. Sports are a social activity and can help you make friends and maintain healthy social activities.

Using Exercise to Effectively Prevent or Relieve Pain

Exercise maintains balance. As we age, our balance gradually worsens. The main cause of poor balance is the loss of feeling in the soles of the feet (neuropathy). Exercise, especially walking, can supply good blood circulation to your feet, which combats neuropathy. Also, exercise helps to improve and maintain your balance because your body must balance itself with each step, thereby allowing your body to the opportunity to use its balancing abilities.

Exercise can prevent many illnesses. Social exercises such as tai chi, aerobics, group exercise classes and dancing can effectively prevent and treat dementia. Exercise strengthens the heart, increases the heart's tolerance to activity and prevents heart attacks.

Exercise can maintain and build up muscle strength and endurance. Beginning at about age twenty-five our muscles gradually weaken, but proper physical exercise can effectively slowdown this process. Regular strength training can improve and prevent the loss of flexibility as well.

Exercise can effectively prevent and treat osteoporosis. Good blood circulation supplies necessary nutrition to your bones and exercise strengthens your bones. I had a patient who took vitamin D and calcium regularly for ten years, but she wasn't physically active. Because of this, she still developed osteoporosis. I suggested to her that if she wanted to have strong bones, she would need to increase her protein intake and exercise more and not just take supplements. Bones are like your muscles in that they need to be exercised regularly. That is why the common saying, "Use it or lose it," applies to exercise and the health of your body.

Chapter Four

Stress and Emotional Health

Learn How to Manage Your Mood & Improve Your Relationships by Improving Your Emotional Well-being

Our mental health and physical health are engaged in a dynamic relationship. Our physical behaviors can affect our mental state. Inversely, and perhaps more importantly, our mental health can affect our physical health. Regardless of how physically healthy a person is, if their mind is not balanced and they are not in harmony with their mental state, they can develop psychological issues which can lead to devastating circumstances and behavior. Balance is as important for mental health as it is for physical health. A balance of both mental and physical health is required in order to be a healthy individual.

Achieving mental stability is both difficult and absolutely necessary in order to be able to lead a satisfying life. Focusing solely on physical health may be easier for some people, but it alone cannot eliminate negative emotions and thoughts. This means that a physically fit person who does not invest in a healthy mind can still suffer from depression, anxiety, anger, fear and other emotional disorders. The mind is capable of changing the habits of the body. Proper education on how to achieve these changes can be the most important tool for leading a healthy lifestyle.

Many emotionally unhealthy problems or activities, such as eating disorders, smoking, alcohol abuse, unprotected sex and drug abuse, are the result of a weak mind. Many people who engage in these types of activities know, on some level, that these are unhealthy, destructive activities, but mentally do not have the capacity to stop themselves. Continuing to engage in these activities continues to weaken their mind, which explains why you may know a perfectly intelligent person who smokes cigarettes. Giving into addiction is one of the most powerful ways to weaken the power of your mind.

When you are able to develop and maintain a healthy mental state, you will be able to make educated decisions concerning the activities you engage in, behavior you exhibit and the choices you make on a day to day basis. You will then be less likely to develop emotional imbalances. Mindfulness, which is to be aware of every emotion and response you experience, can help you control which actions and thoughts receive your attention and energy. Mental wellness is becoming more and more of an important issue in the pursuit of overall well-being and health. Focusing on developing strength of mind may be the most important and life changing thing you can do for yourself. Here are some important areas where the circumstances and surroundings of your life may interact, interfere or improve your mental health.

Diet and Emotional Well-being

Parents know that babies stop crying as soon as they are fed; diet clearly affects our peace of mind. Babies and children cry, are fussy or are difficult when they are hungry, or, in more severe cases, have a nutritional deficiency. Different foods can affect mental states as well. For example, when a child eats too much candy he may become very hyper, restless or unable to focus and then may experience a crash in energy. Sometimes when we are sad or in a bad mood we feel as though certain treats make us feel better (such as the stereotype of eating ice cream after a break up), but, usually these foods have adverse effects due to sugar and fat content. As adults, we are better at hiding our emotions, but maintaining a healthy diet still greatly influences our mental state.

Eating and drinking are natural joys of life. When we are hungry, food is satisfying and tasty. When we are thirsty, water is pleasant and refreshing. However, we should enjoy food and water only when we are hungry or thirsty. It is important to eat regularly throughout the day, but you should really only be eating when you are hungry. If you are not hungry at the time when you usually have a meal, then don't eat a full meal.

You should always take your time and enjoy your food. It is very important to focus on what you eat in order to make sure that you chew your food properly. Chewing is the beginning of the digestive process. The more you chew your food, the easier it is for your body to digest. Taking your time to eat and enjoy your meal is both physically and emotionally beneficial. Unfortunately, because of the modern lifestyle, many people eat in a hurry, talk, argue, fight, read and watch TV during a meal, all of which are horrible for digestion.

Many people fear gaining weight or feel that they need to lose weight, so they eat food that is tasteless and marketed as low calorie food (for example frozen "diet" meals), whereas it is far more nutritious to eat fresh food in portions that are right for your individual body. Poor eating habits can seriously affect your mental health, and are among the main causes of depression in the modern world.[1] When people eat too many high calorie foods (such as fast food) for comfort or pleasure, they consume more calories than their body needs. Overconsumption of food can cause weight gain and obesity, which can cause emotional disorders. Extra fat can make people lethargic, lazy and unenergetic. A whole slew of body image issues usually accompanies the accumulation of weight, which causes the loss of self-esteem, depression and various physical health problems, which can, in turn, cause more emotional problems. You must develop the willpower to control yourself, moderate what, how much and when you eat.

Sustaining hunger for extended periods of time or not taking in enough calories can cause fatigue, depression, insomnia, sleep disorders, body shakes and aches, headaches and fainting. An ancient Chinese saying says, "If you eat until the belly is full, then you will have less homesickness." Many people get agitated when they are hungry; this usually dissipates once you have eaten. Not eating enough of the right kinds of foods can cause nutritional deficiency which leads to health problems that can cause emotional disorders. Many people who suffer from chronic emotional disorders may see a change in their mental state by simply changing their diet and eating habits.

Food can be addictive. We usually crave strong tasting foods that are high in calories, such as meat, cheese, seafood, cakes, etc. The higher in calories a food is, the more delicious and complex taste it contains, which makes it more addictive. It is natural to gravitate towards high calorie foods and it is part of our survival instinct to want to "store-up" energy from food when it is available. Hundreds of years ago meat was used to quell hunger for multiple days. Meat still fills this need for many people around the globe. Meat can sustain us longer than other foods. Considering the modern lifestyle, in which there is little physical movement (unless you exercise), it is clear that we do not need nearly as many high calorie foods as our ancestors. When you want to eat something that is strongly flavored, such as greasy, sweet, spicy or sour food, be sure to limit your intake and be aware that these are addictive types of food. It is true that a high-protein diet can increase your energy and excitement, relieve depression, increase your self-confidence, combat fatigue and increase your tolerance to cold. But, eating an amount or type of protein that is not right for you may increase your levels of stress, anxiety, anger or restlessness. Consuming low calorie foods can increase feelings of calmness and well-being, but if not balanced with other types of foods, it can increase fear, sadness, low energy and low self-confidence.

Being able to enjoy your food and eat healthily (with balanced nutrition) is a sign of self-control. We are confronted and tempted with unhealthy food everywhere, from school and work to the grocery store. Remaining aware that eating unhealthy food can damage your health and can cause an undesirable mental state can help you make the right diet choices. Some people know what they should eat but cannot control themselves. This results in eating disorders, such as obesity (when unhealthy food is eaten in excess), anorexia (when little to no food is eaten) and bulimia (when binging and purging gives the illusion that you can eat whatever you want but, in reality, no nourishment is taken in). Eating disorders are usually the result of mental issues; therefore, successfully overcoming these disorders requires the assistance of a skilled therapist.

The majority of Americans drink coffee. Coffee increases your alertness and makes you feel awake. However, caffeine works, not by giving you energy, but by blocking the neuroreceptors in your brain[2] so that they cannot receive the message that you are tired. Caffeine can cause energy "crashes" later in the day, which may lead to fatigue and headaches.

Alcohol abuse has a serious effect on our mental health. Alcoholic beverages are not unlike narcotic drugs. In fact, before modern drugs and anesthesia, alcohol was used as an anesthetic for surgery. Moderate consumption of alcohol can increase excitement, make us talk or laugh more, decrease inhibitions and can temporarily relieve depression or sadness. The overconsumption of alcohol (alcohol abuse) can cause emotion disorders such as excessive laughing and crying. Emotional exaggeration and overreaction and can cause physical effects such as dizziness, blackouts, poisoning and even death. Drinking too much alcohol may lead someone to engage in unintended or unprotected sex, drug abuse, criminal mischief or even serious misconduct such as drunk driving. Long-term alcohol abuse results in alcoholism, inability to function according to one's own morals, irresponsibility, social issues, separation or divorce, family conflicts, and can cause attention disorder, memory loss and dementia.[3]

Sleep and Emotional Well-being

The quality and quantity of your sleep has a huge influence on your mental health. Many emotional disorders are accompanied by sleep disorders. Again, we can see the root of this in babies and children. When they are tired or sleepy they become fussy or cranky. As adults we may be better at coming up for reasons as to why we are upset or in a bad mood, but, many times, the reason simply is that we are not getting enough good quality sleep. Lack of sleep affects the quality of your mind and your ability to grasp reality. Lack of sleep can impact your emotions resulting in drowsiness, poor memory, poor decision making, attention disorder, depression, sadness, anger, anxiety, body aches and headaches. In fact, insomnia is the main syndrome of schizophrenia, especially in younger people.[4] Good quality sleep relieves mental stress, heightens positive emotions, relieves negative emotions, increases energy, memory and efficiency of work or studying and can effectively prevent mental disorders. Sleeping too much is often a sign of depression, and can cause fatigue, drowsiness, low motivation and poor eating habits.

Physical Exercise and Emotional Well-being

Physical activity affects mental health. Sports can be entertaining. Playing them can be very enjoyable. Playing sports is a good social activity and provides practice and training for developing healthy social skills. A healthy social life is a very important part of maintaining good mental health. Spending too much time alone can cause you to pay too much attention to certain thoughts. Exercise can relieve stress accumulated from work, school or your family. Exercise balances brain endorphins and body hormones, which can effectively prevent and treat emotional disorders. Sports may effectively treat ADHD,[5] build your tolerance to stress, and –the most important benefit –maintain your physical health, which is the basis of mental health. However, improper exercise can affect your mental health negatively. Exercise can be very addictive, especially extreme competitive sports. If you get to the point where you need to reduce or stop playing sports because of health problems or injuries and you find that you do not have the willpower to stop, then you have developed an unhealthy attachment to sports.

Sports physically wear and tear your body, so at a certain point or age, the risk of injury is more of a concern than the potential health benefit. At this point, you should reduce or stop playing these sports. Exercise and sports should be done for health benefits only. If you play sports for money, a scholarship, because you are addicted to the feeling or to show off you can actually increase your stress level and potentially cause more harm to your body than good. Some sports, such as ski jumping, motorcycle or car racing, rock climbing and jumping, parachuting, bungee jumping, etc. are exciting because they raise your adrenaline levels. This is why people who participate in these kinds of sports are often called "adrenaline junkies." They are addicted to the high feeling achieved through raising the adrenaline level in their bodies. I have seen patients who have broken bones because of these activities, but they still cannot stop doing them. Daredevil behavior that causes you to pursue an activity for the feeling, regardless of the costs, demonstrates a weak mind and might even be a sign of a deeper emotional issue.

Chronic Pain Can Affect Your Long-Term Emotional Well-being

Because physical health is intimately connected to your mental health, it should come as no surprise that chronic pain or illness can have a serious effect on your mental well-being. Suffering long-term from health problems can cause chronic fatigue, depression and fear. If you have a chronic health issue, make sure to do as much research on it as possible, and investigate all the potential reasons you may have developed this pain or illness and what you can do to remedy it. You can learn to treat and manage your problems at home. For example, when your blood pressure, blood glucose or cholesterol level is high, you may feel anxiety and may find yourself getting angry easily. But, if you change your lifestyle or take medicine to treat these problems, you will notice that you may feel calmer. If your blood pressure, blood glucose or cholesterol level is low you may feel fatigued, depressed and fearful. If you treat these problems, your emotional health will respond accordingly. Seek assistance from a mental health professional or physician if you think that your mental well-being has diminished. However, if your physician does not inquire as to the cause of your mental disorder, he may be quick to prescribe pills to relieve your symptoms without fully understanding your individual needs. Often times, medications are not properly prescribed and may actually worsen your condition. Actively participate in your health care so that your individual causes of illness and specific needs are properly addressed.

Hormone disorders can seriously affect mental health. For example, females who have PMS or menopause syndrome often experience anxiety, depression, irritability and anger. Many of my patients who have hyperthyroid disorders often complain about emotional disorders and having short tempers. Depression can be a sign of thyroid disorder.[6] Brain injuries or illnesses can cause emotional disorders such as multiple personality disorders.[7] Cancer patients, especially late stage cancer patients, usually are fearful, angry or depressed. Many times, the emotional stress from having cancer can cause the death of a cancer patient before the actual cancer does. One patient of mine had esophagus cancer. He was a construction worker and worked hard physically. He went to the hospital during his lunch hour because of a burning pain he felt when he swallowed food. He had no other physical discomfort. After the doctor diagnosed him with cancer, he had a "meltdown" and died a month later. It was the stress that killed him. Theoretically, he could have survived three more months with just IV support. This demonstrates how powerful the mind is. If you mentally give in, then your chance of survival is slim. But, if you stay mentally strong and positive, you have a better chance of eradicating cancer. The key is to educate yourself about actively preventing cancer. If you have already have been diagnosed with cancer, find the right kind of help or treatment (which is not always the mainstream pharmaceutical approach), build the physical, emotional and medical support system that you need and stay mentally strong.

Anxiety, anger and stress can cause insomnia and can raise your blood pressure. Depression can change your appetite, sleep schedule, cause you to lose your motivation to exercise and take care of yourself, and can, in extreme circumstances, lead to suicide.

Stress can lower your immune system functioning, which allows infections to develop more easily and lowers your ability to fight off common illnesses. When you experience too much mental stress, simply trying to fight off a common cold may overburden your body. Stress is the main cause of shingles outbreaks, hormone disorders (especially for females), irregular menstruation, lack of milk production for a nursing mother and hair loss in men and women.

The Effects of Your Social Life and Family on Your Mental Health

Depending on your family and family history, you may be more prone to mental health issues. Family members are some of the only people we interact with consistently throughout our life; therefore, they have the capacity to affect or influence our behavior. People who grow up in a loving, compassionate, kind and peaceful environment will most likely raise their family with the same qualities. A person who grows up in a violent, abusive household will most likely carry on those negative qualities when they start their own family. These are learned behavioral patterns that require cognitive and intentional habit changes.[8]

Parents - Parents are responsible for loving and raising their children. Nowadays, there are many resources available to help us properly train and teach our children important skills, knowledge and values such as manners, morals, healthy hobbies, habits & behaviors, beliefs and love. What we do and how we act as parents has a profound effect on our children; everything you do or say can influence how your child develops. The more quality time you spend with your children in positive activities such as exercising or playing sports together, spending time outdoors, having good conversations and demonstrating genuine interest in their thoughts and desires, then the more mentally stable they will be.

If you experienced a bad childhood or bad parenting, it is extremely important that you work through the issues you may have developed from those experiences. You must learn how to forgive and forget, so that you can let go of those problems and not act in the same negative way towards your loved ones. For example, many alcoholics claim their drinking problem is hereditary, because their parents were alcoholics, but this is no excuse to continue abusing alcohol. If you want to lead a healthy lifestyle, you must take responsibility for yourself and learn to live healthier and better than your parents did.

Siblings - A relationship with your sibling is a good way to develop social skills and can end up being a very important part of your social life, especially in sparsely populated areas. Siblings can affect your mental health. If children are mean to their siblings through physical or verbal abuse, the victimized or attacked child may have developmental issues or mentally develop slower. Parents must be fair and make sure to watch and teach their children how to get along with one another by engaging them in conversation about their issues with one another. Siblings should respect each other and never take advantage of a sibling's love. Remember, siblings are friends for life, if they are open with one another then their relationship throughout their lives will only grow stronger and be more harmonious.

Spouse or Significant Other - Your partner is perhaps the person closest to you, so your happiness can be more affected by this person than by anyone else. Of course, fighting and arguing is never conducive to a loving environment. Communication between one another is the key, if you are upset about something, you should take the time to a have an honest discussion about it. Never try to solve the issue with yelling or passive aggressive behavior.

Teachers - As children, we spend most of our time with teachers. Teachers should be aware of how influential they can be in a child's life. Teachers help shape the worldviews of children; therefore, they have the responsibility to teach them how to think for themselves, to question everything, to learn how to research and investigate whatever interests them as well as teach them the power of knowledge. It is important that teachers exhibit behaviors, responses and emotional regulation that exemplify self-control and understanding of emotions.

Friends - There is an old Chinese saying that says, "Whatever color paint you use is the color you will get on your clothes." How your friends act and behave will have a direct influence on how you behave. We don't always have control over who we become acquainted with, but if you see that a person pursues negative paths or routes you don't intend to take, then do not create a deeper friendship with them. Having close friends that you can confide in and discuss your problems with can help you to manage stress and help you build a strong, positive support system.

If you are experiencing issues at home, with your family, at work or school, try to talk to a close, trustworthy friend. This may help you relieve stress and may prevent issues from getting worse. Talking to a counselor or seeking professional relationship guidance may be beneficial as well. Overall, good social skills and a good social life can be very beneficial to your mental health. It makes it more difficult to focus your attention on your negative thoughts and helps you enjoy yourself through conversation and the company of others.

The Effects of Natural Disasters and Tragedies on Mental Health

Natural disasters and tragedies can have an impact on a person's mental health, both short and long-term. These experiences can affect your sleep and sometimes even make appearances in your dreams. Such tragedies include death of a close family member (such as spouse or loved one, parent, child, sibling), sexual abuse, war, job loss, physical or verbal abuse, lawsuits and legal problems and serious health problems (such as cancer, paralysis, paraplegic, blindness, etc.).

Take as many measures as possible to prevent the same tragedy from happening again. Use your experiences to help others heal. You may find that sharing your experiences will others will not only help them, but will help you heal as well. Use the law to protect yourself and reprimand the people who have harmed you. But remember, forgiveness is an empowering experience. Forgiving other people helps you let go of the incident; therefore helping you think about it with less animosity or hatred.

Count your blessings. In the case of disasters, it is a miracle that you have even survived. Be grateful in the present moment. Don't let feelings of guilt, confusion or worthlessness take away from the quality of your life in the present day. Stay busy. The busier you are, the less time you will have to think about the tragedy.

As time passes, your memory of the tragedy will become less acute, and you will naturally think about it less frequently. Time is usually the only thing that helps ease the memory of a tragedy. Talk to your friends and family members for comfort. It is very likely that a professional counselor or therapist will be necessary, especially if the tragedy is followed by thoughts of self-harm or suicide. Never hesitate to seek help. Stress, grief and mental health issues are not shameful. Talking to a skilled, professional counselor may be the healthiest and most beneficial thing you can do for yourself.

Drug Abuse and Emotional Well-being

It is no secret that drug abuse can cause severe damage to your physical health, but the damage can be just as bad, if not worse, to your mental health. Drug abuse can cause a multitude of problems, including a family financial crisis, divorce, neglecting or negatively influencing your children, loss of trust, sleep disorders, loss of family and friends, job loss, memory loss and criminal behavior. These issues can act as catalysts for emotional disorders such as depression, anxiety, anger, thoughts of suicide, etc. There are proactive things you can do to prevent the chance of you or your loved ones from developing a drug addiction.

Educate Yourself About the Negative Consequences of Drug Use

Seek out information and learn as much as you can about the physical and mental effects of drug use. Some people get hooked on illegal drugs because they do not understand the extent of the risks they are taking, with both their health and the law. Discuss the potential health, social, legal and mental dangers of illegal drug use with the people you love.
Do not spend time with people who take illegal drugs, even occasionally. Persons with drug addictions are often unpredictable and sometimes dangerous while under the influence of drugs.

Parents –although you cannot control your children –you can show approval when your children spend time with a friend that you feel is a good influence, and communicate your disapproval when they pursue friendships with those you feel may be potential drug users. The absolute best thing you can do is to sustain trust and honesty with your children. If they feel comfortable and safe talking with you about drugs and those who may be on drugs, then you can calmly explain to them the facts about drug use. Don't react in anger when your children come to you for guidance and support. Provide a safe environment for them to share their feelings with you. Establishing and maintaining an open and loving relationship with your children may prevent them from turning to bad influences (like drugs) for comfort and acceptance. Children are often greatly influenced by their parents, especially if they know that their parents have high expectations for them to meet. Be honest and cultivate honesty in your children. Children who are raised to be honest are less comfortable lying about or hiding their drug use.

Take pride in having strong moral and health standards. Understand that you have the freedom to do whatever you please, but certain activities do not measure up to how you would like to treat yourself and your body. Respect yourself by protecting your health. Remember, that even things that may be legal, such as smoking cigarettes or drinking alcohol, have been known to lower inhibitions and lead to drug use, unsafe sexual activity and poor decision making, such as driving drunk.

Many drugs are addictive from the start; therefore, it is best to never try them –not even once! Many people think they can control themselves and will be able to quit when they need to, but desire for getting high again can overpower your will.

If you or someone you love needs help with a drug addiction, seek the help that you need from professionals such as counselors, rehabilitation and detox centers. Ask your family and friends for support, but it is very important to stop drug use under the supervision of a trained professional because quitting some drugs "cold turkey" can lead to serious and immediate health issues including seizures and sudden death. People who need to quit drinking alcohol often need and benefit from professional assistance as well.[9]

Medications and Emotional Health

Some medications may help your physical state, but they can have severe side effects on your mental health; even medications that are supposed to help with mental issues can have severe side effects and can be highly addictive. Here is some information about how different types of medication can affect your emotional well-being.

Antidepressants - are the third most prescribed medicine in America. About one out of every ten people in the United States takes an antidepressant medication.[10] They can be helpful in extreme cases, but the majority of doctors who prescribe them do not investigate whether or not aspects of your lifestyle may be causing your depression. General practitioners are the most likely to prescribe antidepressants, not physiatrists and other health professionals. If you are experiencing depression or other emotional disorders, work with a professional counselor. Taking medication without counseling is irresponsible. Not only is this an irresponsible approach, but many times the medication prescribed to treat your depression can cause more psychological problems, including side effects that can cause physical health problems. Many antidepressant medications are addictive and are accompanied by withdrawal syndrome if you try to stop. Instead, ask your doctor to help you understand what is causing your depression and what kind of therapeutic and alternative treatments may help you.

Because of all the side effects (both known and unknown), medication should be used as the absolute last resort.

Painkillers or narcotics - these medications have a similar effect on your body as heroin does; after all, they are both opiates.[11] These medications can cause fatigue, memory loss, poor memory, drowsiness, attention disorder, sleep disorders, emotional disorders and behavioral problems. They are very addictive, and many people who are given painkillers for pain or an injury often continue taking them after they are no longer necessary. Withdrawal syndrome from painkillers and narcotics includes shivering, heart palpitations, insomnia, severe anxiety, restlessness, body aches, cramps and seizures. Long-term mental effects include insomnia, depression, attention disorder and poor memory.

Sedatives or sleeping pills -these medications are also addictive and can cause fatigue, anxiety, hypersomnia, fear and depression. They can cause physical health problems that eventually affect mental health. Unfortunately, these medications —antidepressants, painkillers and sleeping pills —are the most popular prescription medications in the United States. In fact, the majority of all pharmacy refills are for one or more of these types of medications.[12]

Antiepileptic, Parkinson medication and psychotropic drugs - these medications can cause drowsiness, depression, anxiety and hallucinations.

Hormone supplements and steroids - steroid intake can cause fatigue, depression, hypersomnia and emotional instability. Thyroid medication is meant to affect your body's thyroid hormone, but highly productive thyroid can cause anxiety and insomnia, while a less productive thyroid can cause depression, fatigue or hypersomnia. Male hormones can increase anger, irritability and anxiety. All hormone medications will directly or indirectly affect your mental health in some way.

Antibiotics - can cause nausea, gas, indigestion and various gastrointestinal problems. Antibiotics work by killing bacteria, but the medicine does not discriminate between good and bad bacteria. Therefore, some of the bacteria necessary for your gut to function normally are killed when you take antibiotics. If you have to take antibiotics make sure to take a high quality probiotic to restore your healthy bacteria levels. Health discomforts caused by taking antibiotics can include depression, fatigue and insomnia.

There is no medication that is completely free from side effects. This means that medications can and do cause physical discomfort, and therefore, can affect your mental well-being. If you notice that you suffer from mental health problems after taking certain medications, tell your doctor and talk about changing medications or find non-prescription solutions for your condition if possible. It is ironic that medications –developed to help us – are actually one of the major causes of emotional disorders and instability.[13]

Weather and Emotional Well-being

Many people find that the weather has an influence on their mental state. Seasonal Affective Disorder is very common.[14] Winters spent far away from the equator mean long, dark nights and extreme coldness. In some areas, such as the Pacific Northwest, the number of rainy days can exceed the number of sunny days in winter. Gray, wet, cold days can trigger negative emotions. Thunderstorms, tornadoes, hurricanes, earthquakes and floods can cause fear, anxiety and depression. Changes in air pressure can worsen body aches and pain and can also negatively affect your emotions. Extremely hot weather can cause anxiety, anger, impatience, insomnia, poor sleep quality and fatigue. If you notice that the weather effects your emotions, remain aware of this fact. This will help you more effectively handle your emotions, and you can look forward to feeling better when the weather improves. Try to stay inside where you can make yourself comfortable. Watch a happy movie or read a book in a temperature suited to your liking. If you suffer chronic depression, you should avoid working graveyard schedules. If you live in a dark, cold place it may help to move to a sunnier location.

Weather changes can stir up negative emotions, but they can also be the source of inspiration for positive emotions. You may feel joyful and happy in the first days of spring, when you see the first flowers bloom and the trees begin to blossom. Taking a walk on a warm, sunny spring day can be such a joy. You can enjoy the outdoors during hot summers by going swimming or participating in water sports. You can delight in being able to purchase fresh, local vegetables and fruits. During fall leaves become vibrant with different colors which create a lovely scene. Snowy winters can dress a gray day with a beautiful, elegant white coat.

After it rains the air is fresh and clean and sometimes rainbows make an appearance. It can be relaxing to watch snowfall and enjoy the peace and quiet it renders. It can be exciting to watch a thunderstorm. A full moon is majestic. Sunsets and sunrises are often awe inspiring. Frogs, crickets and birds provide natural music that can be comforting and relaxing. You can train your mind to enjoy any season or type of weather by focusing on the beautiful aspects that each season has to offer. Unfortunately, many people tend to be too enthralled with videogames, TV and computers to be able to take the time focus their attention on the beauty of nature in order to combat seasonal mood changes.

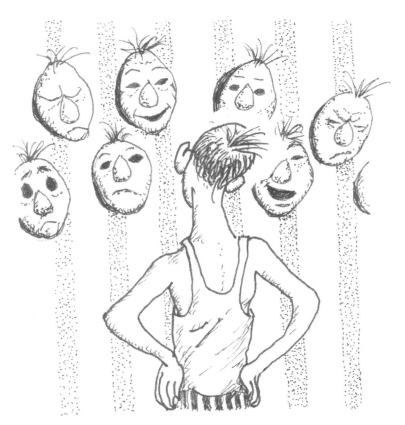

Only you can manage your emotions.

Managing and Controlling Yourself

We often talk about how to discipline our children, students or employees, but, rarely do we ever talk about how to discipline ourselves. It takes great skill and control to manage your own emotions with genuine care and attention. This skill can take a lifetime to learn. Having control of oneself is a sign of maturity, mental health and balance.

We are faced with decisions about how we are going to live our lives on a daily basis. Making the decisions that are best for you and those around you requires a thoughtful pursuit of balance.

Intimacy and Emotional Well-being

Being in an intimate and loving relationship is a joyful part of life. However, engaging in unprotected sex or having too many sexual partners can spread STIs (sexually transmitted infections), which can cause serious health problems and emotional trauma to both yourself and your partner or future partners. Some people feel pressured to have many sexual experiences, especially teenagers and young adults, but these sometimes impersonal sexual relations can cause emotional trauma, especially for teenagers and young adults who may not have the coping skills, self-esteem or maturity to handle these types of impersonal, yet often emotionally-stirring encounters.

Pornography and sexually-themed entertainment –in all of its forms –is somewhat dangerous to emotional well-being. The majority of people who pursue these activities are males, and it can cause them to have unrealistic expectations of their sexual experiences with their partner. This can lead to discontent and can be very offensive to a person's partner. Pornography and sexually-themed entertainment can become very addictive because it provides such an easy way to achieve sexual pleasure. In fact, some men who become accustomed to viewing these intense images find it difficult to perform without the stimulation these images provide. If you want to have a healthy sexual relationship with your partner, I suggest you seriously limit (or altogether avoid) your exposure to pornographic material and sexually-themed entertainment in all of its forms. If you feel that you have a sexual addiction, you may need to seek help from a specifically trained, professional counselor to help you overcome your personal concerns.

Being in a relationship or falling in love is a beautiful experience, but heart break can be devastating and is known to trigger depression, anger, suicide and murder. Maintaining a successful relationship takes hard work, commitment, honesty, proper motives, concern and compassion for the other person. Needing or wanting someone else to make you happy or fill a void that you have in your personality is not a healthy way to enter a relationship. Remember, love is a learning experience; with each relationship, gain knowledge that will help your next relationship be healthier and more successful.

The Effects of Television

Television programs can be very entertaining and educational. The majority of people enjoy watching TV, but spending too much time watching TV is a big problem in the American lifestyle. The average American spends more than five hours a day watching television.[15] Television takes away from family time, causes neglect of children, encourages laziness, reduces use of your mind, discourages physical movement & exercise and can make you crave food when you are not hungry (usually unhealthy foods like chips and soda). Many television programs contain emotionally traumatic content, such as murder, kidnapping, rape, sex, ghosts, etc. News can be very depressing; if you dwell on what you hear in the news, the world can quickly become a negative place. Additionally, TV has many commercials that try to convince you to buy things you cannot afford or do not need. Commercials for fast food or chain restaurants can make food look appetizing, but they all hide how unhealthy these foods are for you. Always question what you hear or see on television, sitting passively and believing everything you hear is just the same as being brainwashed. You need to sustain an active mind by reading, having conversations, writing, playing music, creating art, thinking for yourself, living by your values, etc.

Television, computer and videogames can disrupt your emotional well-being. Many people spend hours in front of the computer reading news, watching a movie, shopping, e-mailing or playing videogames. Most of the news reported is bad news, but we are curious to know what is going on in the world. However, you should never seek out traumatic news because it can cause traumatic shock. Negative news, movies (including the portrayal of anger, fear, violence, murder, sadness or promiscuous sex) and videogames (with sexual or violent themes) can create unnecessary anxiety. The more time you spend engaged in viewing negative images on news reports, movies and videogames, the more likely it will be for you to have a negative emotional response to them, even if you are unconscious of the effects it has on you. Spending more time in front of the TV will increase your risk of becoming depressed, not only because of the content you will view on the television, but also because sitting for a long time will reduce circulation to your brain and cause your mind to become more static. Spending less time on the computer or in front of the television can help you develop closer relationships with your spouse, children and the rest of your family and friends. The more time you talk with your spouse, the more you can enjoy each other's company and communication, and the closer you will be. Arguments and misunderstandings are less likely to occur if you communicate on a regular basis. If you take the time you usually spend watching television and devote it to cooking a healthy family meal or exercising you will become healthier and happier.

Exercise and Emotional Well-being

As I have already discussed, regular, moderate exercise is crucial for good health. Staying dedicated to a schedule or routine makes exercising regularly much easier, and, after a couple weeks, even enjoyable. Exercise is a great way to alleviate mental stress and is frequently prescribed for a wide variety mental health disorders. Exercise builds confidence and self-discipline and promotes a healthy esteem of self and body as well. Developing a healthy view of self through exercise can help reduce mental stress and disorders. You can come up with many excuses as to why you don't want to exercise, but these excuses stem from a lack of willpower. Stay strong and committed to your exercise goals.

The Effects of Sleep on Your Emotional Health

Quality sleep is absolutely necessary for good mental health. An unregulated sleep schedule can lead to staying up late due to spending too much time online or watching TV. This can disrupt your schedule because you will feel tired in the morning, may cause you to sleep during the day and prevent you from feeling tired at night. "Night owls" may claim that they feel best late at night, but this may be because their sleep cycle has been disrupted for a long time. When you cannot discipline yourself to go to sleep when you should, it is more difficult to get up and operate efficiently during the day. This will push the activities you need to do during the day into the evening, encouraging you to stay up late to accomplish the things you need to do. This will prolong the cycle. The inability to function well during the day can lead to negative thoughts and depression. Also, sleeping too much (more than nine hours as an adult) or too late in the day can cause lethargy and can be a sign of depression or other mental disorders.

The Workplace and Your Emotional Health

Work is rewarding and joyful if you love what you do. The ability to sustain a job can be a sign of a responsible, mentally stable and strong individual. You should choose a profession that you enjoy; but, even if you love what you do working too much can cause problems. It can cause you to lose valuable family time, exercise and quality sleep. Stress from work can be detrimental for your mental and physical health, so you must balance how much time and effort you invest in your job.

Daily life is a balancing act based on moderation. In order to establish a healthy day to day routine, you need wisdom and willpower. Each day brings new issues. When you are faced with unpredictable factors, it is important to be able to calmly approach them by remaining in control of your behavior and maintaining your healthy lifestyle. When you can respond well to unexpected elements of life, you can remain in control of your emotions and mental well-being.

The Effects of Stress on Emotional Well-being

One of the greatest enemies of a balance life and well-being is stress. Stress can cause serious physical health issues, as well as depression, anxiety, nervous breakdowns, insomnia, nightmares and suicide. Inversely, the utter lack of stress can cause depression, insomnia and fatigue, as well as memory loss and dementia. So, the goal is not to rid ourselves of stress completely, but rather learn how to manage stress. If stress levels are increased in moderation, the mind has the ability to adapt, adjust and build up tolerance to stress.

Good vs. bad stress –good stress (such as falling in love, nervousness before a social event, preparing for a vacation, winning a contest, etc.) can be very exciting, but can cause anxiety and insomnia. If you experience good stress in high levels too often, your health can be affected by the disturbance in, or lack of, a normal daily routine. Bad stress (such as lawsuits, divorce, job loss, bad health, loss of a loved one, traumatic life events, etc.) has serious effects on mental health, such as insomnia, fatigue, anxiety, anger, depression, even suicide or murder. If you suffer from high levels of stress, you should try speaking with your friends or family about it, or consider seeing a therapist about how to balance your stress level. More neutral emotions (such as normal daily life routine without anger, fear, ecstasy or hysterical emotions) help us feel mentally balanced. You can achieve this state through talking to somebody about your stress (so as to relieve yourself of your worries), writing about how you feel, taking a casual walk, listening to calming music or doing a short breathing meditation.

Lack of stress –without stress we begin to fall apart. In order to stay physically healthy, our body and mind need to be used ("use it or lose it"). For mental fitness, you should stay busy through working or reading. When you have too much vacant time, you may easily develop depression. Older people, in particular, should heed this advice. Although you may have retired, it is good to keep busy; without small goals on a day to day basis depression and dementia can sneak up on you.

Work-related stress –a little bit of stress at work can inspire you to get things done. But, too much work-related stress can cause you to become a "workaholic" or dislike your work, which is very bad for both your mental and physical health. Try to schedule in a relaxing activity every day, even if it is for just fifteen minutes. If you work hard, try to match it with a similar level of playing hard.

Stress Can Be Addictive

Stress and fear stimulates the adrenal glands and the production of brain endorphins.[16] These chemicals have an effect on how we feel. This is why people can enjoy watching scary movies, or feeling fear from dangerous activities like riding motorcycles, rock climbing, parachute jumping, ski jumping or car racing.
We feel anger when we have physical or verbal conflicts with others. Many times we first experience this in our family. The feeling of releasing anger can be addictive because it stimulates the adrenal glands and launches us into a stress reaction. Many people do not know how to communicate properly or how to express their negative thoughts and emotions without arguing or fighting. After conflict, they feel

better and relieved (from a reduction in physical and mental stress), which is why some families may fight on a daily basis. Once you get used to the emotional release that comes after arguing, you will feel uncomfortable and nervous when you do not argue or fight with others. Anger can raise your blood pressure and, in extreme cases, can trigger a heart attack. In a fit of anger, you can make bad choices and can lose control of yourself and your actions. Many people regret the decisions they make or hurtful things they say when they are angry. Anger can be managed with professional help and, in many cases, is necessary for people with anger issues.

Love is a positive feeling. Loving someone or being loved feels wonderful and is a valuable part of a successful social life. Through experience and accumulation of wisdom we learn how and in whom to invest our love. For example, some parents try to control their children, supposedly out of love and protection, but this usually results in a poor or broken relationship with their children.

Almost everybody has been, or will be, in love at some point in their lifetime. Sometimes, you get so addicted to the feeling of being with the person you love that you can hardly function without them. This is not a healthy partnership, but rather an attachment to the feeling of love. When you experience heartbreak from this type of relationship it can be particularly difficult to get over because you crave the feeling associated with being in love. It is important to educate yourself through books or therapy on how to regulate your emotions in any type of relationship.

Depression is particularly dangerous because it is very difficult to recover from. The reason for this is that once you are depressed, even for a relatively short time, you become accustomed to and create a habit of being depressed and eventually become addicted to negative emotions and thoughts. Depression can be a normal reaction to heartbreak, loss of a loved one, painful health issues, etc. Everybody experiences depressive states throughout life. But, if you are depressed often, or if it is the main emotion you experience, you may need help. You know yourself and your life the most intimately. Only you can help yourself by inquiring as to what may be the cause of your depression. You can seek the answers to you the causes of your depression with a skilled and properly trained therapist or counselor.

Ways to Increase Your Tolerance to Stress

Everyone manages stress differently. Each person has their own tolerance for the amount of stress they can handle in their life. However, you can build up your tolerance to stress so that you can handle it better.

Work-related stress –from a young age, children in Asia are taught to study hard. The better scores they get on their final high school test, the better college they can choose. So, children learn to work hard and experience a lot of pressure. Their stress levels reach the highest when they are in high school, college or begin working. However, the stress from work never exceeds the stress they experienced in their youth because they have already learned how to manage stress. But, in America, children have a relatively happy and easy schooling experience. Many have no stress from school, but when they go to college, they have to study hard and make a living to support themselves. Suddenly, work stress has a dramatic effect on them. Many people who cannot handle this stress eventually become depressed. If children are trained at a young age to work hard, then they can build up their tolerance to stress, and therefore, can handle it with greater ease when they are older.

Sports and exercise –can build up tolerance to physical and mental stress. Playing sports can create stress. It is not unusual for an athlete to lose a night of sleep before a major competitive game. While playing the game, athletes are under a high amount of pressure, which can be heightened by the competitiveness of the game. Therefore, a good athlete is not only in great physical condition, but, in terms of stress tolerance, is in great mental condition.

Individual differences –each person's ability to tolerate stress depends on the person's education, upbringing, background, culture, personality and health condition. For example, how a person's family tolerates stress can determine how that person will deal with stress. Because different cultures and religions have different moral standards, (a joke that may be funny to you can be extremely disrespectful to others). Some people have a hypersensitive personality and so it will not take much to upset them and encounter the boundaries of their tolerance to stress, whereas others have an experienced social life, so it takes a lot to offend them. People with health conditions such as those with hyperthyroid, PMS, bipolar disorder and schizophrenia usually tolerate stress very poorly.

Exposure to other people's stress –people's tolerance to stress can change when they are under the influence of illegal drugs, alcohol or medicine and if they do not feel physically strong (if they are hungry, tired or ill). For example, some people tolerate stress better after they take antidepressant medications or narcotics. Some people become angry easily after they have drunk alcohol. If you are aware of how different substances and physical states can influence a person's ability to handle stress, then when you have a situation in which you have to deal with a stressed person, you will be more understanding, thus, able to have a calmer attitude and make it a less stressful situation for everybody.

Age –we experience a lot of stress in life. Our tolerance to it naturally increases as we gain experience and wisdom. As we age, we naturally became more experienced with emotional trauma. Young people, especially teenagers, tend to be constantly stressed because they are, for the first time, dealing with conflicts on their own, which can make them very sensitive and emotional. This can make dealing with teenagers very difficult, but parents should understand their children need space as well as an open ear for help and support in dealing with emotional stress.

When you are under direct verbal or physical attack –we are social beings and in our modern life we are constantly dealing with people (especially in big cities). It is impossible to avoid interactions; you are bound to have conflicts with other people. It is important for your health to cultivate the ability to handle these unpredictable stressful situations safely.

Education and upbringing –the more educated a person is, the more confident they will be. Humility and confidence can help you deal with conflict gracefully or avoid it altogether. Depending on how a person is raised, they may seek out stressful situations or simply ignore issues. Examine yourself and imagine how you would theoretically like to handle a potentially stressful situation and whether or not this is actually how you would handle it. If the two do not match, then think of some ways to remind yourself, throughout the day, how you would like to deal with conflict and how you can change your reactions to match your personal expectations.

Life experience –the more practice you have in dealing with stressful situations, the more wisdom you will gain. For example, people who were brought up in smaller cities or the country may have less experience dealing with stress than those who grew up in a big city. This is because you interact with more and different types of people more often in urban areas. The more you deal with people, the more conflicts you will have, and the more experience you will gain. There are different kinds of emotional trauma (such as physical violence, verbal abuse, relationship problems, work issues, legal issues, etc.), and although someone may be experienced in one area of dealing with stress, it does not mean that they will be able to effectively handle other types of stress. If you find yourself experiencing unfamiliar stress, you can always refer to how you dealt with other kinds of stress in the past and apply your coping mechanisms to the new situation.

The Effects of Emotional Trauma

When people experience severe emotional trauma, such as verbal, physical or sexual abuse, they most likely will develop a severe defense mechanism when dealing with any type of emotional stress. The mechanisms vary. For example, somebody who was physically abused and has become very sensitive emotionally may threaten an aggressor in any type of conflict with legal action, call for law enforcement or even become physically aggressive. As another example, if someone was sexually abused and embarrassed about it, that person may become withdrawn and not open to talking about any emotional experiences.

Often times, the stress of an emotional trauma can cause anger, anxiety and depression. The first step is to communicate about the emotionally scaring situation with a therapist, counselor or a friend you can trust. If you have thoughts of suicide or harming another person, then you must confront the emotional pain with a mental health professional who can help you cope with the damage and learn how to heal and move on.

Test yourself. Imagine the following situation. You are driving improperly and you offend somebody else in traffic. The man honks at you and makes an offensive gesture. How do you react?
1. Laugh at him and think that is he overreacting.
2. Apologize to yourself and feel bad about having made a mistake.

3. Ignore him or pay little attention to the interaction.

4. Honk back and respond with an offensive gesture as well.

5. Pull the car over and get out of the car in preparation for a physical altercation.

6. Speed up, rush in front of his car and slam on your brakes, potentially causing an accident.

If you chose 4, 5 or 6 then you are not handling this kind of stressful situation healthily. Emotional reactions caused by anger or irritation can cause more mental stress and may be a sign of emotional immaturity.

How to Know if You Have a Mental Disorder

Depression, anxiety, anger, stress and feeling worried are all part of normal daily emotions. If you feel negative emotions once in a while, you are probably reacting normally to daily stressors. Serious mental health issues are usually accompanied by one of the following symptoms.

1. If you feel depressed daily or depression constitutes a large percentage of your daily emotions and affects your daily activity, then you may have a mental disorder.

2. If you experience a noticeable personality change. If your friends or family members tell you that you are harder to deal with or you have been acting differently (for example, you used to be outgoing, but now have social anxiety or are afraid of people), then you may want to see a mental health professional.

3. If you have a sudden change in your moral standards. If you start engaging in illegal activities or begin doing things that are against your own moral standards (such as stealing, using drugs, drinking alcohol excessively, missing or being late for work, failing to take care of your family or children, have thoughts of suicide or harm to others), then you need to make an appointment with a mental health professional.

4. Change in your health and personal care. If you gain a large amount of weight, stop taking care of a physical health problem (such as if you have diabetes, but stop managing it or if you have emphysema, but keep smoking), have extreme changes in your eating habits or if you stop taking care of yourself (such as if you were neat and become very

disorganized or if you stop taking showers), experience drastic dress or grooming habits (such as extreme hairstyle changes or excessively tattooing or piercing yourself in a short period of time), if you begin drinking excessively or start doing anything to get high (such as inhaling aerosols or other fumes), then you may have an emotional problem and should see a professional health counselor.

5. If you develop a sleep disorder. Experiencing frequent nightmares, anxiety, low energy, chronic fatigue, chronic drowsiness, insomnia or a sporadic sleep schedule may be a signal of the possibility of an underlying mental disorder.

6. If you experience extreme changes in your appetite or if you have little to no appetite because of stress, depression or an existing eating disorder, you must speak to a health care professional immediately.

7. If you lack motivation to perform daily tasks or to enjoy life. If you cannot find motivation to do anything, especially exercise, consider seeing a mental health specialist.

If you feel that you are suffering from a mental disorder, the first step is to balance the various elements of your life through changing your lifestyle. You can try to address the potential cause of your mental imbalance by speaking with trusted friends or family members, but it is best to seek help from a mental health professional.

Controlling Your Emotions

Emotions are perhaps the most personal things we have. Sometimes, people feel like they are being preyed upon by their emotions, but the reality is that we always have a choice with our emotions. We can choose which emotions to focus on and feed. If we choose negative emotions, then we will become more negative and depressed. On the other hand, if we choose to focus on positive emotions, then we will feel better. We have the power to decide how much an emotion can bother or disturb us. This is a skill that takes great wisdom, knowledge, experience, self-discipline and self-control, but is extremely necessary for dealing with our emotions, especially when extreme circumstances arise in life.

Train yourself to look for positive things in every situation. For example, if it is raining, you can think about how the rain is relaxing and soothing, how it washes the dirt off your car and washes away dust and pollution particles in the air so that the air is nice and fresh after it stops raining. If you focus on these positive aspects instead of the negative ones, like the fact that you cannot go outside or that the sky is dark and gloomy, then your day will be far more enjoyable and the rain will not affect you as much.

Many people like to gossip about others. While it is fine to talk about other people, it is never good to speak negatively about your family members, workmates or friends. Focusing your energy on positive things will cultivate a positive environment around you and a good attitude within. This also reassures you of the positive relationships you have in your life. Talking negatively will create negative emotions and sour feelings, which can lead to weaker relationships between you and those you know. Positive words increase your energy level by making you happy and excited about your life and the relationships you have, whereas negative words do the opposite.

The most important thing is to try and cultivate a positive environment around yourself by doing one or more of the following activities: playing or listening to uplifting music, enjoying social activities with friends, hosting a party, going to party, visiting or talking with a friend, keeping in touch with old friends, playing cards or chess or developing a hobby (such as sewing, knitting, drawing, painting, gardening, handcrafting, etc.). It is absolutely imperative that you eat right and maintain a balanced sleep schedule. Wake up at the same time every day and follow a routine that will motivate you for the day ahead, such as enjoying a relaxing breakfast, stretching, reading inspirational materials, etc. Create a schedule for yourself full of enjoyable activities so that you have several positive events to look forward to throughout the day. By creating a positive environment you can train your mind to pursue the enjoyable aspects of life, and therefore, be a more content person.

Managing Anger

Anger is a normal emotional feeling. Everybody experiences it every now and then. Remember, however, that when you become angry you make the choice to become angry. Instead of having an immediate emotional response to an irritating or frustrating situation, why not first examine what is happening and decide how you would like to responsibly and calmly respond. If you encounter a person who is eager to be provoked, do your best to not instigate the person. If you do not give the person the reaction they are seeking, they may lose interest in pursuing an argument or fight with you. Sometimes it is better to not respond to or walk away from a person who is visibly agitated.

Anger can become an addictive habit. The more often you get angry, the easier it is for your anger to be triggered. If you experience anger daily, it is absolutely necessary to see a specialist, especially if a lack of anger or argument makes you anxious or depressed. For example, I used to have a neighbor who fought with her husband every day. Then, her husband had to leave town for a month. My family and I thought she would we be happy to be alone, but surprisingly, she became depressed. She ended up telling my mother that she felt better after she argued and she needed it to feel satisfied. Clearly, anger was an addictive habit for this woman. If you have anger or arguments daily with your family or friends, then you should consider ways to change your habit. It may be best and necessary for you to receive anger management or family counseling.

Anger can trigger hormones (endorphins) that influence the brain, like alcohol, drugs or medication.[17] Most verbal and physical abuse, violence and other crimes are carried out under the influence of anger. Often times, when people have calmed down and have cleared their minds, they usually regret their anger driven behavior. In the end, anger ends up hurting yourself and your relationships more than anything or anyone else. If you often feel ashamed of how you act under the influence of anger, then you have an anger problem. There are many books and articles available online and at the library that discuss how to manage anger. Look for tools and wisdom from whatever sources you can find to help you address this issue, however, it is best to seek help from a professional counselor who is experienced in anger management.

Anger can be heightened when we are under the influence of different substances. Alcohol, drugs, narcotics, hormone medications and substances naturally produced by our bodies all have an effect on how we tolerate angering situations or emotions. For example, some people remain relatively calm while others become very angry when under the influence of the chemicals produced by stress, physical health problems, hunger, extreme temperatures and fatigue.

Managing Depression

Depression is also a normal aspect of emotional feelings. Our modern lifestyle has made depression more common and causes it to occur more frequently. If you are depressed, the first thing you should do is figure out what is the cause of your depression. Pay attention to your daily routine and your lifestyle and see which activities are followed by a depressed state. For example, eating low calorie foods can cause you to be more lethargic which leads to less exercise, which can make your more prone to depression. You may also be going through certain experiences, such as relationship or life changes that can be difficult to accept. But, resisting the changes will only deepen your depression. This is why it is important to observe and accept the events in your life. Only after this step can you start to make changes in how you interpret your situation. Also, keep in mind that often times we can only see the good of a situation after some time has passed. It may take you a couple of weeks or months to see what you have learned and how you have actually benefited from what, at first, seemed to be a depressing experience. If you keep this in mind, then you will be much less prone to falling further and further into depression. Of course, as already discussed, it is often best to talk to a counselor or therapist as you discover and work through the cause of your depression.

Skills to Help Manage Your Depression

Because depression is a normal part of our mental activity, there is no real way to cure it and ensure it will never return. You will always have low and high moments in life. It is important to be mindful of what you are experiencing and not get too attached or overly affected by any one state of mind. A helpful practice is meditation. Through meditation you can calm the mind and devote time to being calm and worry free. Eventually, you can start to incorporate meditative states into your everyday life.

How to Meditate

Most people sit up with their legs crossed and their back completely straight with their hands gently resting on the knees. This is a popular image of being in a meditative state. However, you may find this position to be uncomfortable at first. You may find that it is best to lie down on the floor or on a comfortable surface when you first begin practicing meditation. You should lie down on your back with your arms resting comfortably with your palms facing up. Your entire body should be relaxed (lying down to meditate is great to do before bed and may help you improve your ability to fall asleep). First, center yourself; make sure that you are sitting or lying evenly so that you are not leaning more to one side than the other. Then close your eyes and your mouth and bring your awareness to your breath (which is being done through the nose). Breathe normally, simply observe your breath. Then, after a couple minutes, try to emphasize your inhalations and exhalations by making them longer and deeper. Make sure that all the muscles in your body and your face are relaxed. It may be helpful and soothing to visualize your inhalation breath coming into your body through your nose, up and down the center of your head and down your spine. You can image your breath moving from the bottom of your spine to the front of your belly and moving up your stomach and through your chest and throat and out through your nose with exhalation. Repeat breathing with heightened awareness for as long as you like, if your mind gets distracted, simply bring your awareness back to your breath. At first, this may be difficult to remember, but keep reminding yourself and it will eventually become natural to you. After you have finished breathing with awareness of your breath and body for at least a couple of minutes (fifteen to twenty minutes is usually a good length, but you can do it for as short or long as you like), then breathe normally for a couple of minutes and observe the differences in your body and the heightened clarity of your mind.

You can take just a few minutes during the day, even if you are at work, to calm and center yourself by focusing on your breathing. You may find that this will energize you, release built-up tension and improve your overall mood. As you progress, you may find yourself enjoying learning new types of meditations, adding soothing music to your mediation time or using guided meditations to help you work through difficult emotional experiences.

Self-Discipline

It takes great willpower to make the right decisions, as opposed to just doing what we want to do. For example, things such as poor eating habits, watching too much television, alcohol abuse, drug abuse and excessive use of medication can perpetuate or cause depression. If you can remind yourself that these bad habits add to your depression, it will be easier to avoid doing them. Breaking these bad habits is a test of determination (will-power). Once you have developed an understanding of how these things can affect your mental and physical health, you will no longer find your bad habits to be attractive ways to spend your energy, time or money. With time, you will find that the positive benefits of following through on good habits will be very rewarding and make it easier to maintain good habits over the long run.

Although antidepressant medication does help many people feel temporarily less depressed –it does not cure depression. In fact, most people who take antidepressant medication continue to suffer from depression.[18, 19] Many people have to take other medications to combat the side effects of antidepressants. The more medicine you take, the more mentally reliant you become on it for general stability. For example, I had a patient who took antidepressant medication, but the medication caused her to constantly sweat. The sweat began to emotionally affect her daily activity, so she went to a doctor for her perspiration problem. The doctor gave her a medication and her sweat was brought under control by the new medicine. However, it caused her to develop dryness, so her doctor gave her medication for dry eyes, mouth, skin and body aches. You never know what the effects of one medication will be on your entire body and eventually your mental health.

Another patient of mine had insomnia caused by antidepressants. When he went to see his doctor about his insomnia, his doctor gave him sleeping pills. After a year of being on sleeping pills, his insomnia worsened. He could not sleep at all without the medication and even found it difficult to sleep when he took the medication. He developed anxiety because of his sleeping issues. His doctor suggested that he take an antianxiety medication. I have seen plenty of patients who have had similar experiences with medications and doctors. It is no surprise that over twenty percent of Americans are taking more than three prescription medications in any given month.[20]

I have several patients who work as registered nurses in various nursing home facilities. These nurses have told me that close to one hundred percent of all of their residents are under orders to take antidepressant medications. It is often easier for elder-care facilities to have their residents medicated rather than address the causes of geriatric depression through positive mental health care and social programs.

Are antidepressants really necessary for the majority of the people who take them?

No.

Are there other, healthier ways for people to manage their depression?

Yes.

Unfortunately, in America, many doctors take the approach that antidepressant medication is the answer for depression. Antidepressant medication should not be the major answer for depression. There is no shortcut or easy way to deal with depression. At first, it may seem easier to simply swallow a pill. But we have to take into consideration other issues –physical and emotional –that often surface with the use of antidepressant medication. It is easy to get addicted to the high feeling taking medication may provide you with at first. For the sake of your health, consider the potential side effects of long-term use of these drugs. Consider all other treatment options available to you.
Is prescribing medication just an easy "quick fix" for you and your doctor? What steps are being taken so that you, your doctor and other healthcare providers (such as your therapist) are working with you to address and treat the underlying cause(s) of your depression? What are your other treatment options? What can you do, for yourself, to relieve symptoms of depression? What interventions are necessary for you to regain emotional control of your life? What lifestyle habits need to be addressed? How can you participate in your care so that you can regain emotional health?

Medication at times is necessary and can provide the intended results. Medication should be the last option for mental health disorders, not automatically the first choice. The main point is that you need to take responsibility for and participate in your depression treatment. It isn't healthy to hand responsibility for your mental wellness and place the state of your emotional well-being completely in someone else's care.

Overall, the key to managing your emotions is to be aware that in your waking state, you have thoughts and emotions –that, unlike during your sleeping state –you have the power to control. Think of emotional feelings as being in three groups: negative emotions (feelings of depression, anger, anxiety, fear, worry, etc.), neutral emotions (feelings that result from doing work, completing your duties and routines, etc.) and positive emotions (the feelings that come from falling in love, playing sports, doing hobbies, taking a vacation, etc.). If you invest your energy in neutral emotions and positive emotions, then you will have less energy to spend on creating negative emotions. Be intent with your emotions and reactions. Be present in each moment. Be aware of and recognize your feelings. Make a conscious choice to protect and preserve your emotional well-being before you respond to events and your environment.

Staying busy can keep you out of emotional trouble. For example, young people who are busy with school or sports will have less behavioral problems and emotional breakdowns.[21] Stay focused on your life's purpose and set goals for yourself. It is important to have goals in your life so that you can work hard to reach them. A goal, in combination with positive, healthy habits, helps create a positive and healthy environment around yourself and in your life. This will lead you to a more stable, productive, happier and healthier life.

Chapter Five

Sleep Management
Better Health through Better Sleep

You will spend more than one third of your life sleeping. Everyone has a bad night's sleep every now and then. Unfortunately, as many as seventy million Americans are not able to get enough sleep on a regular basis.[1] Sleep disorders have different causes which will be explained later in this chapter. However, good sleep along with a proper diet can help remedy almost any sleep disorder and help you feel rested and energetic throughout the day. Once you are able to determine which type of sleep disorder you have and which of your existing health conditions are contributing to your sleep disorder, you will be able to take preventative steps in order to resolve your sleep issues and achieve quality sleep.

Seven Most Common Forms of Sleep Disorders

Inability to Relax –some people find it very difficult to fall asleep because their minds stay active and alert, so they spend hours tossing and turning in bed before being able to fall asleep.

Inability to Fall Asleep or Stay Asleep –some people may be able to fall asleep quickly, but they may wake up a few hours later and find that they can't fall back asleep. Other people may not be able to fall asleep at all, even though they feel tired and do not have anything on their minds that is keeping them awake.

Inability to Stay in a Deep Sleep –some people have no problem falling asleep, but because they are light sleepers, they are awoken by the slightest sound and are unable to achieve deep sleep. People with this type of sleep disorder often find it very difficult to function in a normal environment because outside noises and noises from other people in their home may prevent them from being able to sleep without disruption.

Sleeping too Much –it is possible for some people to sleep more than they need. Sleeping too much can prevent your brain and body from getting the oxygen and nutrition it needs. This can cause you to develop chronic fatigue and organ damage.

Snoring –some people snore or have untreated sleep apnea. These people constantly wake up throughout the night and feel tired during the day because they did not get the deep sleep their body needs.

Lethargy –some people frequently complain that they feel tired, drowsy and sleepy or that they simply do not feel well. Lethargy is a form of exhaustion that can affect you physically and mentally. Temporary exhaustion may be a normal result of working too much or too little, jet lag, depression or too much or too little activity. It may be a sign of mineral or vitamin deficiencies as well. Temporary exhaustion is common when a person is fighting an illness such as a cold or infection.

Lethargy may affect a person similarly to the way alcohol does. A person who is lethargic may have reduced cognitive ability, reduced alertness, inability to perform simple tasks, etc. A person suffering from lethargy shouldn't drive a car because their ability to focus and react is greatly reduced.

While short-term lethargy (fatigue) is normal and happens to everyone at some point, chronic lethargy is a serious health concern because it can slow down your metabolism (because of reduced energy level), reduce your motivation to take care of yourself and increase your risk of developing high blood pressure, diabetes and high cholesterol.

Some common causes of feeling chronically fatigued include obesity, poor lifestyle habits (such as not scheduling enough time for adequate sleep), insomnia, side effects of certain medications (especially antianxiety drugs and sleep aids), side effects caused by being physically or mentally ill, brain injuries (such as stroke, tumor, infection, dementia, etc.), illnesses, jet lag, lack of regular & quality sleep and old age.

Hypersomnolence Disorders –some people suffer from disorders that affect their ability to sleep well. These include narcolepsy, sleep terrors, sleep apnea syndrome, talking while asleep, sleep walking and grinding teeth at night. These disorders commonly cause a person to develop lethargy as well.

Hypersomnolence disorders may be genetic, but for the most part, their causes are not well understood. However, it is possible to manage these conditions and possibly reduce their frequency. The most important things you can do to reduce these disorders include preventing overtiredness, overstress and emotional overstimulation. Extreme emotions such as anger, excessive laughter, sadness and fear can trigger or worsen hypersomnolence-related syndromes.

If you currently have a hypersomnolence disorder, avoiding alcohol and drug use and maintaining a regular sleep and work schedule can reduce the frequency of your syndrome and lessen your sleep disruptions.

How Sleep Disorders May Negatively Affect Your Health

Fatigue –low energy, drowsiness, inability to concentrate, body aches and pain can all be caused by even a small amount of sleep deprivation. Long-term sleep disorders can cause fibromyalgia or involuntary nerve disorders. Fatigue and low energy can lead to low motivation to take care of oneself and can affect organ processes.

Metabolism –sleep disorders can affect your metabolism and cause you to gain weight, elevate your blood pressure or increase your cholesterol levels.

Lowered Immunity –lack of sleep can decrease your stress tolerance and reduce the functioning of your immune system; making it easier for you to get sick and harder for you to recover from illnesses. That is why rest and sleep are the most common doctor's recommendations for recovering from illnesses.

Emotional Disorders –sleep deprivation can lead to emotional disorders. For example, children become cranky when they do not get enough sleep. Adults do not cry or act out in the same way as children, but it is clear that at a very primal level, the amount of sleep you get can affect your emotions. Stress management can be difficult to achieve when you have a sleep disorder. Sleep disorders can cause physical and mental health problems to develop or worsen. Likewise, existing health or mental problems (such as depression) can make it even more difficult to achieve good quality sleep.

Attention Deficit and Memory Problems –a night of lost sleep can prevent you from being able to concentrate on tasks or remember what you need to do throughout the day. That is why it is commonly known that drowsiness can increase your risk of being involved in an auto or work-related accident. The attention level of a tired person is equivalent to the attention level of someone who under the influence of drugs or alcohol. Long-term sleep disorders can increase your chances of developing dementia later in life.

Health Problems Can Cause Sleep Disorders Body Aches & Pain or Fibromyalgia –can affect your quality of sleep by keeping you awake or consistently waking you up throughout the night. If you suffer from pain, body aches or pain or chronic pain conditions such as arthritis or fibromyalgia, you need to pursue effective preventative treatment to resolve those conditions. Itching is also considered to be a type of pain. For sleep health, it is particularly important to treat and prevent itchy skin.

Asthma, Cough or Congestive Heart Failure –are health problems that can affect your body's oxygen supply. Lack of oxygen can cause nightmares, reduce your ability to achieve deep sleep and cause you to wake up frequently throughout the night. Coughing is an irritation that can prevent you from being able to even fall asleep.

Anemia –can cause heart palpitations, which can cause you to develop anxiety. Acute anemia caused by heavy menstruation, childbirth or donating blood can cause sleeplessness as well.

Unbalanced Glucose Levels –too high or too low glucose levels can cause sleep disorders.

High or Low Blood Pressure –blood pressure that is too high or too low can seriously affect your ability to fall asleep, stay asleep or achieve deep sleep.

Hormone Disorders –can seriously affect your ability to get a good night's sleep. Almost all hormone imbalances cause some type of sleep disorder. For example, hyperthyroidism can cause severe insomnia. Menopausal syndrome and post-operative hysterectomy problems can cause sleep disorders because of the imbalances these cause to your hormones. Different hormone disorders can affect your ability to sleep in different ways, so balancing your hormones properly can help improve the quality of your sleep and may even eradicate your sleep disorder.

Emotional Disorders –depression, anxiety, stress, fear and other emotional disorders can cause or worsen sleep disorders. Some people develop sleep anxiety as children and never outgrow it. Some people suffer from anxiety, stress or fears that prevent them from being able to fall asleep. Some people are afraid of the dark or to sleep alone, even as adults. Some people have concerns and stresses from life events that prevent them from being able to achieve a good night's sleep.

Urinary Disorders –prostatitis, frequent urination, overactive bladder, incontinence and urinary tract infections can prevent you from being able to achieve a good night's sleep and may worsen any existing sleep disorders you already have.

Stroke –can cause sleepiness. It has been my experience that stroke patients can fall asleep quickly and often and have trouble staying awake. This is because stroke can damage a person's brain. This brain damage can cause sleep disorders such as hypersomnolence disorder, snoring, sleep apnea, lethargy, etc. Once your stroke has passed the acute stage, you should not over sleep (more than eight or nine hours a day) because too much sleep can cause your brain and body to lack oxygen and nutrients and slow down your recovery. Addressing sleep disorders should be an important part of a stroke rehabilitation plan.

Snoring –occurs because the wind pipe is obstructed. This is essentially the same as being subtly choked while you sleep. Snoring can raise blood pressure, can cause heart problems and can even cause sudden death. Sleeping on your back, being overweight, lack of or overdoing physical activity, chronic rhinitis, head colds, tonsillitis, brain damage and reduced brain activity caused by sleeping pills can all increase your chance of snoring.

It is important to find the cause of your snoring and address it. Do not ignore it because of the potential health concerns snoring can create. Some people find that CPAP machines help relieve their snoring. In some cases, because the potential health risks may be considered serious, surgery may be appropriate and necessary in order to relieve snoring.

Medications –when taken to treat certain health conditions and ailments, certain medications can adversely affect your ability to achieve quality sleep or may cause you to sleep too much. Most medications, over-the-counter or prescription, are chemical compounds that affect the body in a multitude of ways. Sleep disorders are just one of the common side effects of many types of medications.
Medications can indirectly and directly affect sleep quality. Narcotics, antianxiety drugs, antidepressants and hormone replacement medications are some examples of medications that can seriously affect sleep quality by causing you to either want to sleep constantly or by preventing you from getting a full night's sleep. If you develop a sleep disorder after starting a medication, be sure to talk to your doctor about it. Sometimes changing medication brands can help address your newly developed sleep issue. High blood pressure medications can disrupt your regular sleep patterns if they cause your blood pressure to drop too low.

Prescription and over-the-counter sleeping pills may seem to help your sleeping problems at first, but can make your sleep disorder worse when you try to stop taking these medications. Some sleeping aids are addictive. It is best to determine what exactly is causing your sleep disorders and address the root cause with preventative care rather than immediately turning to sleeping pills to temporarily solve your sleep issues.

How Much Sleep Do I Need?

One of the most common questions my patients ask me is, "How long do I need to sleep every night?" The average adult needs to sleep approximately eight hours a day. Some people think that the more you sleep the better. But sleeping too much is actually detrimental for your health. When asleep, the body's blood circulation slows down, which can lead to a lack of oxygen and nutrients for your brain and body, thereby making you feel more fatigued when you wake up. Sleeping too much can cause involuntary nerve disorders. Some people may sleep for an adequate amount of time, but don't experience good quality sleep. For example, snoring can prevent you from achieving deep sleep. Determining whether or not you get enough sleep is dependent on the quality of you sleep achieve as well as your individual health conditions. Regardless of how many hours you sleep, if you wake up feeling energized as opposed to tired throughout the day, then you are most likely getting all of the sleep you need. Remember, it is not just the

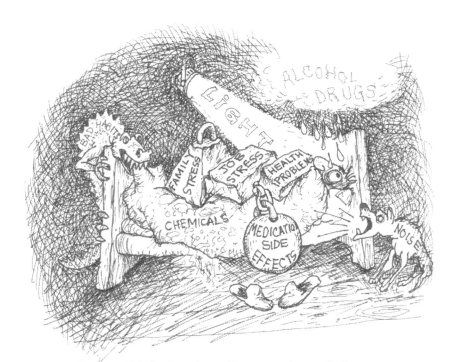

Do you think sleeping pills are going to help you if you don't address the reasons you can't sleep?

quality of sleep you get; it is also important to get enough of the quantity of sleep you need. Having a short, deep sleep will not make up for long-term lost hours of sleep.

Lifestyle Habits and Your Environment Can Affect Your Ability to Achieve Quality Sleep

Most sleep disorders are simply the result of bad sleeping habits. In other words, most people do not take the need for getting enough good sleep seriously and, therefore, do not schedule enough time into their day to get the sleep they need. They allow themselves to develop bad sleeping habits, such as going to bed late. Many people completely disregard the importance of good sleep, so at bedtime they engage in other activities, such as watching TV, playing videogames, reading or surfing the internet. These people are called "night owls". They often feel less energetic during the day, but get more energetic as evening approaches. They either do not have a complete understanding of their biological needs or don't have a strong enough will power to control their behavior. Unfortunately, these people often rely on coffee or energy drinks to get going and keep energetic throughout the day. It is important to go to sleep at around the same time each day and to factor in enough time to get all of the sleep you need. *Use your life clock to go to sleep and wake up naturally.* If you keep a routine, then you can go to sleep even when your body doesn't feel tired. Sticking to a daily routine will make it much easier to fall asleep, help you achieve good sleep quality and can make it easier to wake up.

Car noise and traffic can disrupt sleep. If you live in a city, it may be difficult to avoid car noise pollution. However, you can install noise proof wall insulation or noise proof windows to help diminish outside noise pollution. If you live in an area with a lot of outside noise, do not sleep with the windows open.

Your partner's or a family member's snoring can be very disruptive. Many people lose good quality sleep because of a partner's snoring and are afraid to offend their partner by sleeping in a different room. But, if your partner snores, then it may be better for your health to sleep in separate rooms.

Make sure your bedroom furniture and door does not make noise when opened or closed. If your partner gets up during the night or gets up before you, then the noise from the moving furniture (such as drawers, closets or even the bedframe) and the bedroom door can wake you up.

Noisy pets can disrupt sleep. Pets often make noises when they want to go outside, be fed or receive attention. If you want a dog and you live in the city, it is best to choose a dog that can stay indoors for extended periods of time and can be easily trained not to bark. Consider your and your dog's needs and health when choosing a dog. Noise from neighbor's pets can also affect your sleep. Noisy barking can be a major cause of tension between neighbors.

Bedroom temperature can affect your sleep. Hot temperatures excite the brain, which can make it difficult to fall asleep. It is important that your body is warm and that your head is relatively cool to help you achieve better quality sleep. People usually have better sleep in cooler temperatures. Cold temperatures make blood vessels constrict and put people into hibernation mode, which causes tiredness. This explains why people tend to sleep more in cold weather and tend to feel more tired during winter days. However, temperatures that are too cold, especially low body temperatures can irritate your body or cause pain, which may make it difficult to fall asleep. Cold temperatures below 40 degrees Fahrenheit in rooms where you sleep can prevent you from being able to fall asleep. Do not sleep next to an open window. Outside temperatures drop during the night and in the early morning, so even though the wind may feel nice at the time that you fall asleep, it is likely that the outside temperature will become too cold during the night. Light sleepers may be disturbed from the sensations caused by cold winds.

It is best for everyone in a family to be on the same sleep schedule. This will prevent the noise of someone getting up and ready for the day from diminishing everyone else's sleep quality. If you must keep different sleep schedules, take precautions to avoid disturbing those who are sleeping if you are awake by not using household items that create noise or produce light. Avoid waking up people in your home so that their deep sleep is not disturbed. This can cause them to be restless and fatigued the next day.

Light in your bedroom can reduce your quality of sleep. The best sleep environment is, obviously, the dark. Darkness in the bedroom creates a soothing, peaceful environment. It is a natural reflex to get tired and go to sleep when the environment is dark. The darker your sleep environment is, the better your sleep quality will be. Eliminate as many light sources as you can during sleep, including glowing lights from alarm clocks and other electronics. Sleeping in total darkness helps your body repair itself while you sleep and may play a role in preventing cancer.[2]

Avoid using loud alarm clocks, computers or other electronic machines in your bedroom. Some people listen to music or leave the TV on when trying to fall asleep; this keeps your senses alert and can disturb your normal sleep patterns.

Fresh air in your bedroom contributes to better sleep quality. A lot of people do not realize how chemicals and pollutants in their home can affect their sleep. After staying in an environment for a period of time, the nose becomes desensitized to continuous or common smells, both good and bad. But you are still breathing in potentially toxic chemicals and pollutants even if you can't smell them. After being breathed in, these substances can get into your blood stream and affect your quality of sleep and, in extreme cases, such as carbon monoxide from burning wood, coal or propane in the home, can even cause death. Also, cooking can pollute indoor air and can cause irritation and inflammation in the respiratory system that can disrupt your quality of sleep.

Before sleep, your mind should be neutral and at peace. Clearing the mind is important to avoid nightmares and achieve deep sleep.

Do not watch scary movies before going to bed. These movies can cause nightmares. Nightmares cause unnecessary stress that can affect your sleep quality.

Manage your emotions before going to sleep. You can learn how to neutralize your emotions and manage them properly. Negative emotions can cause sleep disorders and, inversely, sleep disorders can cause emotional problems. It is important to openly work through emotional problems so that they do not resurface in your dreams.

Lying down to think before going to bed is a bad habit. Although lying down helps circulate blood to the brain and can help clarify thoughts, it is best to avoid doing this before going to sleep for the night. Thinking about or planning for the next day can put stress on and excite the brain which can make it difficult to fall asleep. My experience has taught me that thinking about the past can lead the mind to a peaceful place, thereby making it easier to fall asleep, whereas thinking about and planning for the future excites the mind.

Short, daytime naps can help relieve lethargy. In some cultures, it is common for people to take a nap in the afternoon. A short nap can effectively boost your energy and make you feel recharged. But, if you do not nap correctly, it can worsen your syndrome. The best nap lasts for about fifteen to twenty minutes. If you nap too long (longer than one hour), you may end up feeling tired or drowsy for the rest of the day.
Taking too long of a nap during the day can affect your ability to fall asleep at night as well. It is best to only take one nap per day. Older people who tend to nap frequently are less able to sleep well at night because their parasympathetic nervous system is worn down by bedtime. This is why sleep disorders are known as involuntary nerve disorders.

Help your children maintain a healthy sleep schedule. You can do this by making sure they have enough time in the evening to get properly ready for bed and are well prepared for the next morning. Develop an enjoyable and loving nightly routine so that your children will be happy and ready for a good night's sleep. Keeping time set aside each evening to get ready for bed will develop a lifelong healthy habit for your children, keep them healthy and reduce their stress. A nighttime routine will reduce or eliminate going to bed stress for children and will allow them to wake up rested and ready for the day.

Prepare for a Good Night's Sleep

By preparing for sleep, you can mentally and physically become aware of your natural sleep pattern and develop a sense of calm and neutrality by consciously emptying your mind before sleep. This can be achieved through meditation. Meditating before sleep can help improve your sleep cycle and may help you achieve deeper and higher quality sleep over time.

Train yourself to develop habits that will help you fall asleep. A regular routine can help prepare you for sleep. Showering, taking a bath, washing your face or meditating can all be helpful ways to prepare for bed. In China, people prepare for bed by washing their feet with warm water. This not only relaxes the feet, but it is also a way to train the body to get ready for sleep.

Do not drink a lot of fluids for at least one hour before going to bed. Extra water can make you too excited and can disturb your sleep. This is especially important for older people or people who suffer from frequent nighttime urination. Do not consume sweet or caffeinated beverages and foods, such as soda, chocolate and coffee in the evening; sugar and caffeine make it more difficult to fall asleep.

Do not smoke or drink before going to be bed. Smoking can excite your mind and prevent you from being able to fall asleep.
Address drug and alcohol addictions. Drug and alcohol addictions can cause severe sleep disorders. See Chapter Nine for more information about this topic.

The time of day that you take medications can affect your sleep. Do not take diuretics before going to bed. In general, it is best to not take narcotics or antidepressants before going to bed. If you are taking these medications and are experiencing sleep disorders, talk to your prescribing physician about changing the time of day that you take your medications.

Do not do extreme or exciting physical exercise one hour before going to bed. However, taking a casual walk, performing tai chi or yoga before going to bed can help maintain good circulation for your brain. Lack of good circulation in your brain can result in light sleep which can cause you to wake up often throughout the night. As people age, poor sleep quality is often the result of poor circulation; doing gentle exercise before going to bed can help combat this problem. For people who wake up after a couple hours of sleep and find it difficult to fall back asleep, I suggest taking a walk, even it is just around the inside of your home, as a way to increase brain circulation.

Do not eat too much at dinner or before going to bed. Falling asleep with a full stomach stretches and tires the stomach because the food does not move from the stomach to the intestines as efficiently as it does while you are awake during the day. Allow at least three to four hours to lapse after a large meal before going to sleep.

Do not go to sleep on a completely empty stomach. Going to sleep with a growling stomach is not good for your sleep quality. So, if you wait a couple hours after dinner before going to bed, make sure to eat a meal that will keep you satisfied until the next morning.

Make sure you can breathe well. Clean your nasal cavity before going to bed and make sure your nostrils are clear. Find out which positions help you breathe the best and try to sleep in those positions. Sleeping on your back, as opposed to sleeping on your stomach, tends to help facilitate nasal breathing.

Find the bed that is right for your health. A well-suited bed is important. A mattress that is too hard can affect your sleep by causing body aches and pain. A mattress that is too soft can affect your sleep by improperly curving your spine, thereby not maintaining the back's natural posture. Soft mattresses can cause or worsen lower back pain, whereas sleeping on a firm (but not too hard) mattress can help relieve and prevent lower back pain. Sleeping on a thin pad, in a sleeping bag or on the floor can cause body aches and pain that may disrupt the quality of your sleep.

Find the right type of bedding for your needs. Bedding can affect sleep quality. Blankets and bedding influence body temperature, which, in turn, affects sleep quality. While sleeping, it is best to have a cool head and a warm body. It is important that your body is covered during sleep; this includes feet, arms, shoulders and neck. Sleeping with parts of your body uncovered can lead to discomfort in those areas. Use the right types of blankets for the different seasons. The best pillows maintain your natural neck posture. Pillows should hold the weight of your skull; the back of your head should rest on the pillow. Pillows that are too high bend your neck upwards or to the side too much; this can affect your breathing and can cause neck pain. Pillows that are too low can cause your neck to bend to one side too much. Some people put a skinny pillow under their neck. But, when doing so the weight of your head is placed entirely on your neck. This can cause neck pain, headaches, breathing problems and can severely affect your sleep. Pillows that are too hard can cause headaches or neck pain.

The right kind of sleepwear is important. In reality, it is best to sleep naked. Without clothes, nothing can constrict circulation while you sleep. Some people like to wear pajamas while they sleep. If you do wear pajamas, they must be loose fitting. Wearing pajamas that are too tight, especially around the waist, can constrict blood circulation, irritate your skin and muscles and cause pain. Some people should wear warm pajamas. For example, mothers who have to get up often to take care of their infants or sick children. Whole body pajamas can be helpful for people who move a lot at night and kick their blankets off or sleep walk.

Choosing the Best Sleeping Position for Your Health

Choosing the proper sleeping position is important for sleep health. Sleeping on your back is the best sleep position because it is the sleeping position that relaxes body muscles, joints and organs the most. Sleeping on your back maintains your spine's natural posture and helps decongest your sinuses.

Back Sleeping –sleeping on your back should be your main sleeping position. However, this position is not best for everyone. When sleeping on your back the tissues above and around the wind pipe are relaxed. This can cause the tissues and muscles around your wind pipe to fall on your wind pipe and cause snoring, which, as I have explained, is deeply disruptive to good quality sleep. While lying on your back to sleep, do not wear heavy clothes or put heavy blankets on your belly or heart; weight on your belly and heart can cause nightmares. If you have heartburn or emphysema, do not lie flat on your back. Elevating your head a little bit can help relieve heartburn and symptoms of emphysema. Pregnant women should avoid sleeping on their backs because this position can cause back pain, reduce the level of nutrients provided to the fetus and other problems.[3]

Side Sleeping –sleeping on your side is the next best sleeping position. If you have hip or shoulder pain, you should not sleep on the side that is in pain because lying on that side can make your pain worse and affect your sleep. If you are over fifty years old it is best to not sleep on your side as your main sleep position because it can increase your chance of having shoulder pain. If you do sleep on your side, it is best to sleep on the side of your writing hand. The muscles of your writing arm are slightly stronger than your other arm, which means they are better able to sustain the weight of your body. So, this means that the majority of people should be lying on their right side. However, if you have TMJ or vertigo related to issues in the right side of your jaw or in your right ear, then you should not lay on the right side of your body. Some people like to curl up in the fetal position while sleeping on their side, but this is bad for your spine. Lying on your left side is generally not good because it puts pressure on your heart, which is constantly pumping. If you have an ear disorder on the left side of your body, then you should definitely not lie on your left side. Pregnant women may find that it is best to sleep on their left side because this may improve nutrient flow to the fetus.[4]

Stomach Sleeping –sleeping on your stomach is the worst sleeping position in most cases. Exceptions include if you are severely overweight, in which case sleeping on your stomach is the position that puts the least amount of pressure on your body. If you have digestive disorders or gas, then sleeping on your stomach can help you pass gas and relieve discomfort. If you have body pain and sleeping on your stomach provides the most pain relief, then it is appropriate to sleep on your stomach. Some people find that they snore more when they sleep on their stomachs while others find that sleeping on their stomachs reduces or eliminates their snoring. If you snore, it is important to figure out which sleeping position reduces snoring for you. If you are a woman, sleeping on your stomach places pressure on and reduces circulation to your breasts, which may increase your chance of developing breast cancer. When lying on your stomach, your face has to turn to one side which means that your neck is stretched.

Overstretched neck muscles can easily cause severe neck pain and headache. Also, due to gravity, blood drains into one side of your sinus cavities when your neck is turned to one side and can cause sinus congestion. Generally speaking, it is best to choose the sleeping position that you find most comfortable and that is most conducive to helping you achieve the best quality of sleep you can. Lying in one spot or position for too long can cause pain because of the strain of body weight placed on that area. Although cuddling during sleep is pleasant, doing so can be disruptive because any movement that your partner makes can disturb your sleep. Also, the weight of your partner's head on your shoulder, or any part of your body, can cause pain and disrupt your sleep.

Arguing or fighting with your partner before bed time can seriously affect your sleep. Talking in bed is a bad habit because it stimulates your brain. If you talk in your sleep, grind your teeth, punch, kick or walk in your sleep, then you need to take measures to effectively treat these problems. Release stress before going to bed. Try to keep a regular sleep schedule. If you or your partner have health conditions that cause sleep disruptions, it might be better to sleep in separate bedrooms so that you don't negatively affect each other's sleep quality. For example, people who have vertigo or emphysema should sleep with a slightly elevated bed, but this does not mean that their partner will be able to sleep well in an elevated bed. Overall, it is important to make the right decisions for both your own and your partner's health. Try to be understanding and help each other achieve good quality sleep.

Regular physical labor and exercise helps maintain good quality sleep. Physical labor causes healthy fatigue, helps to balance endorphins, maintains good circulation and effectively detoxifies your body. However, not all exercise is good for sleep. Extreme exercise, like marathon training and running, can make it difficult to fall asleep. Stress related to extreme exercise and competition can make it difficult to fall asleep as well.

Achieving good sleep is not only very important to maintain your health, but being able to sleep well is a sign of being in good health. Healthy sleep will assist in keeping your nervous systems properly balanced. Sleeping too much or not enough can be a sign of poor health and of an unbalance system (body). Do your best to maintain a high quality of sleep so that you can maintain a high quality of health.

Chapter Six

How to Create a
Healthy Living Environment

Our modern lifestyle, especially over the last fifty years, has created more and more environmental toxins and pollution. It is impossible to escape being exposed to pollution in form or another in today's world. Today, there are about 75,000 chemicals used in production commercial in the United States and of these, about 30,000 of these chemicals are used commonly.[1] Unfortunately, the majority of the population is becoming more and more accustomed to living with chemicals in their lives, and are willingly adding chemicals to their lives. I would say that most people today are chemical happy, that is, people prefer the smell of chemicals than of natural odors. People consistently choose chemical products over natural products because of their convenience and fast-acting results without taking into consideration their long-term effects. This is often due to a lack of knowledge or understanding about just how toxic these products are. Another consideration is that people often choose chemical products because of the cost associated with using natural products. Most people do not fully grasp the consistent concentration of chemicals that they are exposed to throughout the course of their day. From our homes to our work environments, from our modes of transportation to the clothing we wear –chemicals are present in almost every activity necessary for modern living. It is close to, if not completely, impossible to escape constant exposure to chemicals. However, there are steps you can take to greatly reduce the unnecessary use of chemicals in your life.

Regardless of what you do or where you go, it is almost impossible to escape constant exposure to chemicals. People put chemicals on their bodies in the form of makeups, creams, lotions, fragrances, perfumes, soaps, washes, etc. People absorb heavy metals and plastics through the clothing and jewelry items they wear on their bodies. People ingest chemicals through supplements, vitamins, minerals, antioxidants, prescription medications, weight loss supplements, protein powders, etc. Additionally, people breathe in toxins from cigarette smoke, landscaping & gardening chemicals, bug sprays, candles, room fresheners, paints, arts and crafts supplies, etc. People breathe in chemicals from furniture outgassing and the plastic-based household products they purchase and use regularly.

People consume chemicals that are used during production of crops and fed to livestock. Commercially prepared food is usually shipped and packed in plastic containers. Plastic containers or plastic coated papers are generally used to serve and store food once it is taken home as well. You can enter almost any retailer and smell the toxic fragrance created by the outgassing of plastics, papers, woods and other chemicals. Factories and production facilities produce environmental pollutants that enter our water, air and food supply as well. Whether you can smell these toxins or not, they are entering your body and they can have an effect on the quality of health you are able to achieve.

Environmental pollution has become a major threat to our health. Respiratory disorders, such as nasal and sinus allergies, asthma and COPD are very common today. The majority of these disorders are directly caused by exposure to environmental pollution. That is why lung diseases are a leading cause of death in the world today.[2] Our lungs must breathe these toxic chemicals into our bodies every day, because of this, these toxic chemicals and carcinogens can enter our blood stream. (Carcinogens can enter our bodies through our mouths by what we eat and ingest orally as well.) These chemicals can cause cancers.[3] This may explain why cancer is such a common disease today. There are ways to use common sense to reduce your personal exposure to environmental pollution.

Air pollution is the main pollution that is present in our environment and threatens our health. People complain about how poor the outside air quality is and how polluted outdoor air is, but most people do not understand or realize that indoor air is usually much more toxic than the air outside. In fact, indoor air pollution is a much larger threat to our health than outside air pollution because indoor air pollution is held in a much smaller space with less clean air exchange or flow. Indoor air pollution adds to whatever outdoor air pollution we already are burdened with. In all likelihood, you spend the majority of your time indoors. You live and sleep in your home. Indoor pollution can affect your health more than outside pollution. You may not be able to control what happens outdoors, but you can control the amount of indoor air pollution you are exposed to in your home. You can change, clean and control the quality of air inside of your home. Here are some tips to improve the quality of the air inside your home that will allow you to breathe healthier.

Cook in a properly ventilated area. Cooking inside your home can create poor indoor air quality. Burnt foods, grease, cooking oils, aromas from spices & produce, gas and wood burning stoves can create a poor air quality environment in your home.[4] It is better to cook outdoors or have a separate kitchen that is built away from your living area. At the very least, it is important to use an exhaust fan that pulls cooking smoke and odors outside. Open windows inside your home while you are cooking to allow steam created from baking and frying to flow outside. Steaming and boiling foods reduces the amount of oil that is burned inside a home, but steam created from these cooking methods still needs to be pulled outdoors.

Limit or avoid using chemically based cleaning products in your home. Cleaning products contain a wide variety of strong and toxic chemicals that can create pollution inside your home. Chlorine bleach, glass cleaners, disinfectants, degreasers, furniture polishes, dusting sprays, floor cleaners, shampoos, conditioners, soaps, perfumes, body washes, carpet cleaners, shoe shining oils and cleaners, pesticides, etc. – whether they smell pleasant or not –can greatly pollute your indoor living environment. You should use as few chemicals as possible (or better yet, no chemicals) to clean your home. Use natural cleaning products (not necessarily naturally-derived cleaning products, but actual natural ingredients that have not been overly chemically altered. The term "naturally-derived" does not always mean that a product does not contain potentially harmful toxins.) Do not keep bottled chemicals inside your home; they should be stored outside of your home in the garage or other storage area.

Limit or avoid using chemically based products on your body. Products can release pleasant fragrances and smells, but just because something smells good does not mean it is good for your health or even safe to use. The majority of cologne, perfume, makeup, shampoo, hairspray, hair color, lipstick, lotion, face cream, tanning oil, sunscreen, nail polish, etc. products contain potentially carcinogenic ingredients, toxic chemicals, allergens, hormone disrupting additives, chemical, man-made fragrances and more.[5] Man-made chemicals are cheap to produce, thus making products more affordable. Chemicals are more shelf stable allowing products to be shipped and stored for long periods of time. (Recently, it has become quite common to find consumer skin care products that have been made in Mexico or China. Products made in these countries are not required to ingredient regulations or manufacturing standards of the United States Food and Drug Administration.[6]) Longer shelf lives add profits for producers because there are fewer wasted goods when products do not spoil.

Because people like to smell good, people usually have a variety of different fragrances they keep in their homes for personal use. Some people are more concerned with looking and smelling good and less concerned with the toxins that are seeping into their skin and blood stream. It is well known that hair color additives contain cancer causing additives.[7] Yet, the majority of people who use hair color prefer the vanity of covering their grays over protecting their health. Looking young has usurped taking care of their health. Either they don't care or they simply haven't taken the time to learn about the potential effects of the products they put on their bodies. Some soaps and facial creams (especially creams designed to lighten the skin) contain mercury.[8] Is any amount of superficial or perceived beauty worth risking your health?

For your good health, the fewer chemicals you use, the better your health will be. Unfortunately, most people in modern life are chemical happy people who like or love these chemicals and claim they can't live without smelling good or using artificial grooming enhancements. Do not be chemical happy. You should choose to use natural products whenever possible. For example, if your lips or face are dry you apply a small amount of organic olive oil or vegetable oil instead of using petroleum-based lip balms or heavily preserved facial lotions. This can effectively keep your lips and face moisturized; and olive and vegetable oils are safe if ingested. You don't want to eat coal or lead so that your lips can appear to be colored.[9, 10, 11] It has become much more common to find home and body products that contain 100% natural ingredients. Plant-based products can often be used in place of perfumes and cleaning agents. However, any scent or ingredient (even natural plant extracts) can be an allergenic or become toxic when not used properly. Chose products that do not add chemicals to your daily routine and that are safe for your entire family to use.

Choose wood furniture. Furniture woods, glues, papers, etc. contain harmful chemicals such as benzene[12] and formaldehyde that can cause some people to develop an allergy syndrome or illness. Formaldehyde is a commonly used additive, yet it is known to be carcinogenic.[13]

Unfortunately, it is very difficult to find furniture made from real wood anymore. Woods are often treated with alcohols, stains and other toxic chemicals. Wood sealers and polishes used on furniture can release chemical pollution into an indoor environment. Try to buy furniture that is made of real wood and that has not been treated. When you polish, wax or condition your wood furniture, choose natural products. For example, pure jojoba oil can be used as an effective, safe and odorless wood conditioner. It may be healthier to buy used furniture because new furniture has to outgas (release into the air) the toxic chemicals that are used in making it. After you buy new furniture (wood or fabric covered), you should let it sit outside (or in your garage) to outgas for a few weeks before you bringing it into your home. This will greatly reduce the amount of toxins you have to live with and breathe.

Your whole home can release chemicals as well. Carpet, drywall, paint, plumbing fixtures, ceiling panels, molding, wall covering, curtains, fabric covered furniture, mattresses, etc. all release toxic man-made chemicals into a new or remodeled home. If you plan to move into a newly built or renovated home, you need to open the doors and windows and let it outgas for a long time before you move into it.

Do not live in a home while it is being remodeled. I had a family of three who were all my patients. Each one was sick with a cough and stuffy nose for about six months. Their doctor had given them all kinds of medicines and nothing had helped them. When they came to see me, I talked to them and I was able to find out that they were remodeling their home and had been remodeling it for the last six months. They had been remodeling one part of the house and living in another part of the house at the same time. I recommended that they open all of the windows and let the house breathe (outgas). I told them that the chemicals from remodeling and the new fixtures were causing their coughs and runny noses. They followed my recommendation and all reported reduced symptoms within a few days and all three were able to recover quickly. You should use your nose and common sense when you feel sick. Remember, the smells created by newly built or remodeled homes can be harmful to your health.

Choose clothing made from natural fabrics and do not use toxic chemicals to clean your clothing. Certain kinds of clothing can pollute your home as well. Today, most clothing contains some amount of synthetic fiber such as polyester and other chemical materials.

Clothing is dyed and often glued or coated and these additives can cause allergic reactions in some people.[14, 15] Clothing that is fragranced from detergents, softeners or other chemical cleaning agents, as well as dry-cleaning chemicals, can pollute your home. If you hang clothing in your bedroom that has been treated with any of these additives, it can cause you to breathe this pollution throughout the night while you sleep and may contribute to respiratory problems and other health ailments.[16] You may have become accustomed to these odors. When you sleep or stay in a room for a while, you may not notice the chemical smells at all. In order to tell just how strong these odors may be in your clothing, go outside and get some fresh air, then come inside and go to where your clothes are hanging and you will be able to tell how strong the smell is. Leather clothing and shoes can release high levels of toxins especially from the protective or shining chemicals used.[17] It is better for you to store these items in an outside space such as your garage.

For your health, don't purchase synthetic materials or have your clothing or household items dry-cleaned. There are other alternatives which are much safer for your health and your environment such as buying clothing made from natural materials and having your clothing items wet-cleaned. Do not use fragranced or chemically based laundry detergents, softeners or boosters. Don't use fabric softeners. Avoid using bleach; if possible use heat temperature to sanitize clothing instead of bleach. Wash your clothes and household items in natural (non-synthetic), fragrance-free soaps.

Dust in your home can be breathed into your lungs and affect your lungs' health and contributes to childhood asthma.[18] Although your nose, windpipe and lungs have a great ability to filter and clean out dust that is breathed in, dust can still be sucked into your lungs.

Where does dust come from? It comes from our dead skin cells, products and chemicals that we use in our homes, animal and pet dander, pollen, dirt and other particles that are come into our homes from outside. You can see from your clothes dryer how much lint comes off just your clothing. You can look at the sunlight to see how much dust is floating in your home. Keeping your living environment as dust free as possible is important for the health of your lungs. Having wood, tile, laminate, etc. flooring instead of carpet can reduce the amount of dust in your home because it is easier to see and remove dust from these types of hard flooring surfaces. Avoid using powdery substances on your body, such as baby powders or fragranced body talc. If the wind is blowing or there is visible dust outside, don't open your windows. Dust and clean your home frequently with a wet towel. (Using plain water or water with a small amount of natural soap instead of chemically based cleaning agents can greatly reduce the amount of air pollution added to your home.) Avoid using feather dusters or dry towels that can cause dust to be thrown back into the air. If you or someone in your family has allergies or asthma, it may be best to not keep indoor pets inside your home.

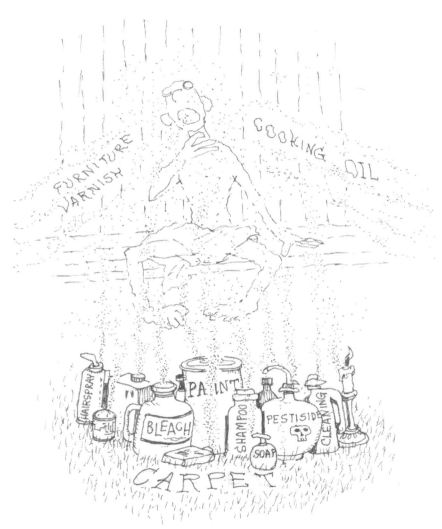

Air pollution isn't just outdoors.

Sources of Outdoor Pollution That Can Affect Your Health

Automobile exhaust is usually the main outdoor pollution source in populated areas. These chemicals are carcinogenic.[19, 20] Take necessary precautions to avoid breathing in these toxins, especially diesel.[21, 22] If possible, avoid living near highly trafficked roads. Don't walk, run or ride a bicycle near heavily trafficked areas or on the side of heavily trafficked roads. Don't spend time near running vehicles or in busy parking areas. Avoid spending time outdoors during inversions or when air quality is poor. Reduce the amount of time you spend driving in traffic and don't drive with your windows open or with your outdoor air vents turned on when you are in heavy traffic.

Burning wood can create outdoor pollution. In the countryside, burning fields, wood, straw, etc. can fill the air with a choking amount of smoke. In the city, burning natural gas, heating oil, coal, propane, etc. to heat buildings can create a tremendous amount of air pollution, especially during cold winter months. If you have respiratory disorders such as asthma or COPD, use extra caution to reduce your outdoor physical activity on days when there is an outdoor air quality advisory.

Farming and landscaping chemicals can create pollution. Products commonly used in farming, landscaping, lawn care, gardening, etc. such as fertilizers, pesticides, fungicides and herbicides not only smell bad but are also bad for your health.[23]

Work-related Pollution Can Affect Your Health

Almost every work environment has some type of environmental pollution. One way or another, you will most likely be exposed to some type of toxin at some point in your life. Since the majority of us have to work and live a contemporary lifestyle, it is generally impossible to avoid exposure to toxins. It is best for our health that we are aware of potential risks and use common sense in order to reduce our chances of inhaling harmful pollution. Whatever you do for work, it is important to educate yourself about any potential toxins used that you may breathe, touch or even consume and the health risks related to these pollutants. Once you have learned the potential risks, you can take the necessary precautions to reduce your exposure to these pollutants by using the proper tools, protections and skills required to perform your duties safely. Be proactive and take the necessary steps to protect your health.

Manufacturing and factory workers are commonly exposed to a variety of pollutants. Products that contain chemical additives or strong-smelling ingredients such as plastics, fertilizers, pesticides, paint, pressboard, shoes, toys, certain foods, etc. all release very strong odors during production and can seriously affect your health.[24] If you work in a manufacturing facility, make sure that the area you work in is properly ventilated and has a sufficient amount of clean air being circulated into the area. Remember, the stronger the odor, the more likely a substance is to be potentially harmful to your health. Use your nose and your common sense to judge the quality of air that you are breathing in. Although your nose can be blind to certain smells that you have become accustomed to smelling, you can always trust your brain use common sense to protect your health.

Retail stores, shopping centers, salons, repair shops, restaurants, and other commercial areas are often full of toxic air. Commercial settings such as nail salons, auto body shops, shoe stores, drug stores, clothing stores, restaurants, etc. usually contain several sources of potentially toxic odors such as wall coverings, carpet, cleaning chemicals, plastic products, furniture, etc. If you work in one of these types of stores, you need to make sure the area is well ventilated. Some people wear masks as a way to protect themselves from the fumes of nail polish or auto body paint, but surgical-type masks are not able to filter out chemicals. They only filter out large particles. If you work in an auto body shop, you should wear a good respirator that can prevent you from breathing in spray paint particles.

I had a patient who started working in an auto body shop when spray painting cars had become very popular. At that time, he was in his twenties and no one wore a mask. No one was concerned or knew that the fumes could be damaging to their health. He told me that he remembered how strong the paint smelled. He worked for some time without any problems. Then, suddenly, he passed out while at work and had to be rushed to the emergency room. The doctors were not able to determine what had happened to him or why he had passed out. So, he went back to work. He passed out again and was rushed to the emergency room two more times before he was able to figure out that the fumes from the spray paint were poisoning his respiratory system. He had been exposed to the fumes for such a long time that he didn't realize the paint fumes were harming him, but eventually, his body built up so many toxins (paint particles in his lungs) and became resistant to the fumes (that contain paint particles) that he could not be exposed to the fumes even for a few brief moments without becoming seriously ill. He had to quit the job he loved. Now in his fifties, he has been suffering from pulmonary fibrosis for thirty years. He can no longer engage in any type of physical labor or even moderately intense exercise. He is extremely sensitive to all types of paint odors and can experience trouble breathing even if he smells paint. If you are a painter or welder, you should stay upwind of your equipment and avoid breathing in toxic smells. If you already have a respiratory disorder, you should consider changing your job.

Repeated exposure to dust or smoke in your work environment can cause illness. If you work in a place where there is a high percentage of dust such as mining, some factories, bakeries, farming, lawn care, etc. make sure to wear the proper mask to protect your lungs from breathing in the dust. Even though your respiratory system has a great ability to filter and clean your lungs, you can still breathe in too much dust because there is only so much your system can handle. If you do not protect yourself properly you may end up with dust-related lung disease (pulmonary fibrosis) which may also increase your risk of developing COPD and lung cancer.[25] If you work as a firefighter or cook, exposure to smoke can seriously affect your health almost the same as smoking cigarettes. You should wear the appropriate mask to protect your health and make sure the kitchen you work in is properly ventilated.

Protect Your Lung Health while Exercising Outdoors

Avoid exercising in areas where unpleasant odors are present. Dust blown around in the air can also affect your health. Try not to exercise when the wind is blowing hard because there will be more dust and pollen in the air. Try not to exercise in a fragrant area or where there are a lot of flowers. Some pollen may smell good, but it is not healthy for you to inhale it, even if you are not allergic to it. Fog is dust that is coated with moisture. It is not healthy to inhale fog. Try not to exercise outdoors on foggy days. Factories, gas stations, restaurants, chemically-treated lawns, housing dryer exhausts, etc. can release harmful pollution. While exercising outdoors, avoid areas where these odors are present.

Overall, if you have a respiratory disorder, stuffy nose, runny nose, sinus pressure, sinus infection, chronic cough, asthma, COPD, etc., especially if the disorder is chronic, you should avoid working in or living near heavily chemically polluted areas. Changing your work or living environment may help to heal chronic respiratory disorders. When choosing a home location, chose areas that are far away from commercial and industrial centers as a way to reduce your exposure to air pollution. Even if you do not have these disorders, you may develop them later on from being overexposed to pollution because chemicals present in the air can get into your bloodstream through your lungs. This is probably one of the reasons why so many people have cancer. If you want to detox your body, one of the best ways to do so is to not breathe toxins into your body. Use common sense to protect your health.

Reduce Your Exposure to Toxins Present in Some Foods

I did not have access to a modern diet when I grew up. I had never seen boxed or packaged food. I had never seen colorful drinks. We ate grains and vegetables that we had grown. We ate fish that we caught or meat that we had raised. But today, in America, food is contaminated with chemicals, pesticides, additives, preservatives, etc. It is then packed in chemically treated papers, plastics and metals, etc. And finally, the food is prepared for consumption by adding more toxins through cooking methods such as grilling, smoking, frying, burning, etc.

For your good health, try to eat more garden vegetables and organically grown produce. At least try to eat fresh foods that have not been boxed, dried, wrapped in plastics, processed, etc. When at home, prepare your food using healthy cooking methods. Avoid drinking water that has been treated with chlorine, fluoride, or other additives or that has been stored in plastic in order to limit your exposure to environmental pollution. Chlorine can be reduced in tap water if the water is allowed to sit out in an open container for a few hours, boiled or filtered. Boiling tap water before drinking it can also kill any potentially harmful bacteria or parasites that may be present in the water. Do not drink water that has been stored in plastic containers, especially if it has been left out in the sun.[26]

Reduce Your Exposure to Noise Pollution

Noise created in the environment can damage your hearing, affect your quality of sleep, add stress to your life and affect your emotions. There are ways to reduce your exposure to noise pollution.

Reduce the Level of Noise Coming into Your Home from Outside. Automobile engine noise or honking can create stress that can affect your ability to maintain a peaceful environment, even while you are inside your home. In order to protect your health, chose a home that is far away from heavily trafficked areas. If you cannot move, you can have insulated windows, sound proof walls or insulation added to your home or areas outside your home to reduce noise from coming into your home. If you live in an area that is close to a busy road, planting trees, installing sound walls or berms may help reduce noise as well. Wearing ear plugs is not healthy as a long-term solution to reducing your exposure to noise because they can irritate your ears leading to inflammation and ear infection.

Reduce music and television volume in your home. Loud music or television is the main noise pollution in a home or car, especially for younger people. Listening to loud music for long periods of time can cause permanent hearing loss. Using earphones for a long period of time can cause ringing in the ears (tinnitus) and permanent hearing loss. I am always surprised by just how many patients I see in my practice that are chronically suffering from ear damage caused by exposure to loud music. Loud music that stimulates your senses can be addictive. Some people become so addicted to noise that they continuously have background noise in their home and may not even be able to fall asleep without leaving the television or radio on. This type of overstimulation can affect your quality of sleep, prevent you from achieving deep, restful sleep and may affect your alertness during the day.

Reduce noise caused by pets. Noise created by barking dogs can affect a peaceful living environment and may cause you and your family to lose valuable rest and sleep. Pets can increase your joy and reduce stress, but choosing the right type of pet for your lifestyle is important. The wrong breed or improperly trained dogs can disrupt not only your life, but the life of your family and neighbors. Barking and unruly dogs commonly cause divisions among neighbors. Before you choose a pet, you should seriously consider not only your needs, but the animal's needs as well. For example, different breeds of dogs have different temperaments. Some dogs are naturally noisier, bark more and are more difficult to train. For example, Chihuahua, Poodle, Terrier and Beagle breeds tend to bark more than other breeds. Before choosing a pet, make sure that you are able to meet the animal's needs and that your home environment is suitable for the breed you have chosen. Make sure that you are able to properly take care of your pet and will be able to meet its needs. This will add to the quality of your life instead of taking away from it.

Reduce noise created by home machinery. Equipment used to make your home a comfortable and convenient living environment such as air conditioners, furnaces, water heaters, exhaust fans, dishwashers, refrigerators, washing machines, clocks, computers, air fans, etc. can also create noise pollution inside your home. The constant background humming created by these machines can disrupt the peacefulness of your home. Look for ways to reduce the noise created by these machines. You may be able to turn them off when not in use or run some of them while you are not at home. Choose the quietest model you can when replacing home appliances.

Chapter Seven

How Temperature and Weather Conditions Affect Your Health

In modern life, with the abundant use of air conditioning and heating and the reduction of outdoor labor jobs, the majority of our daily activities take place indoors. Most of us work indoors, travel in cars and have very little need to be outdoors for more than a few minutes each day. Even the majority of exercise takes place indoors. Because of this, the weather has had less of an impact on our day to day activities and most people don't pay attention to weather changes that are not considered extreme weather conditions. It is true that it is less likely than before for weather to disrupt your daily activities, but weather can still affect your life and your health.

Exposure to Cold Temperatures Can Affect Your Health

Regardless of where you live, the weather, especially exposure to cold temperatures, can affect your health greatly. Even so, different cultures think differently about the effects of cold weather and how exposure to cold affects your health. In Chinese culture, exposure to cold temperatures is considered "an invasion of cold evil" (creating a negative impact on health) and is the most likely of all the weather conditions to negatively affect your health. That is why the Chinese encourage each other to dress warm and to eat warm foods. But in Western culture, people don't mind being cold as much, and certainly do not take into consideration that exposure to cold can be a large factor in the decline of their overall health. In fact, in Western culture, most people do not believe that exposure to cold temperatures can impact their overall health. It is often claimed in the United States that it is impossible to catch a cold from being cold. As you have already learned, I do not agree with this concept. Exposure to cold greatly reduces your immune system's ability to fight off infection, thus, being cold increases your risk of becoming sick because your body is less able to fight off illness. I believe that when you are cold your body's immune system is taxed by having to work harder to maintain your body temperature. This lets your body's "guard down" so to speak, allowing foreign invaders, such as cold and flu viruses, to escape the notice of your immune system; thereby making it much easier for you to get sick when you are cold. Weather changes make it easier for you to get sick as well because your body simply isn't prepared to maintain your internal body temperature when exposed to rapid changes.

Different people are able to handle tolerance to cold differently. Some people enjoy being cold, while other people are sensitive to being cold or simply can't tolerate being cold at all. For example, some people with Raynaud's syndrome physically change color when they are exposed to cold. Regardless of your personal tolerance to cold, there are facts about being exposed to cold temperature that you need to understand in order to protect your health.

Cold can lower your immune system's ability to respond to invaders. It is easier to get an infection or worsen an existing infection when you are exposed to cold. That is why when people get respiratory infections caused by a virus or bacterial infection they say, "I caught a cold." Or, "I have a cold." When the weather changes, especially when large temperature drops occur, (when you're not prepared and have not worn the proper protective clothing), you will easily catch a cold. It has been demonstrated by Eastern and Western culture and is even true for animals.

Some of my patients who are professional cattle ranchers have told me that they can anticipate whether or not their herd is going to become ill based on shifts in weather temperatures. If the temperature experiences a large drop overnight, the ranchers have to go out and check their cattle and often end up treating their cattle with antibiotics to reduce the effects of pneumonia. Interestingly, this happens usually during the first weather change of the season. Some of my patients have told me that when they have placed their sick calves in a barn as a way to keep them warm, they have noticed that their calves have recovered from being sick faster than when they have kept their calves out in the cold weather. Some of my ranching patients have asked me why their cattle get sick more often in autumn than during the coldest part of winter. I tell them that it is because their cattle grow thicker fur for insulation over time while they are exposed to cold weather and become more able to tolerate exposure to cold. In autumn, the temperature changes quickly, so their cattle have not had time to adjust their ability to tolerate cold. They still get sick with pneumonia in winter more often than during spring and hot summer though because the outside temperature during these months is much warmer and less taxing on the cattle's immune systems. When a person has been stranded outdoors in cold temperatures or in cold water for a while, they will have developed a fever and cold syndrome by the time they are rescued; this is another example of how exposure to cold can weaken the immune system. If you dress appropriately for the outdoor season and prepare for possible sudden weather changes, then your chance of catching a cold will be reduced. This is a thousand years of Chinese medical experience; at least, it has proven to be true and work for me in my experience.

Cold can irritate your respiratory system. Exposure to cold can cause you to develop a runny nose or worsen your existing runny nose syndrome. People with asthma or COPD often notice that their symptoms get worse during winter. Also, their chance of catching pneumonia is much higher in winter. If you dress warm and stay indoors, you can relieve your syndrome or prevent it from worsening.

Cold can negatively affect your cardiovascular system. People with high blood pressure are more likely to be affected by exposure to cold. I have learned through my practice that the patients I have seen with high blood pressure tend to spend more time in areas where there are cold winters and relatively cooler summers. I have also seen a tendency for heart attacks and strokes to be more common during winter than summer. If you have high blood pressure, you may notice that your blood pressure is elevated during winter months. If this is so, then it may be necessary for you to talk to your physician about having the amount of medication you are taking adjusted to keep your blood pressure lowered during the cold of winter. Keep in mind that it is important to dress and stay warm during winter as a way to help reduce your risk of heart attack or stroke.

Cold can reduce or slow down blood circulation in your joints. That is why people who have MS (multiple sclerosis), RA (rheumatoid arthritis), lupus, etc. feel more pain and stiffness in cold weather. Dressing warm will reduce your exposure to cold during outdoor activities and can prevent joint pain and stiffness. Cold can affect your skin's circulation as well. Your skin becomes drier in cold weather. People with chronic dermatitis will notice that their syndrome worsens during winter. Dress warm or apply a natural protective oil (such as olive oil) to relieve dry, itchy or cracked skin that can be caused by exposing your skin to cold air.

Weight gain can be caused by living in colder climates. Most people gain some weight during winter because cold temperatures weaken people's motivation to be active and increases people's appetites. Many people think that it is natural to put on a few pounds for protective insulation during cold weather. Also, it seems that people and animals that live in colder climates are generally heavier than people and animals that live in warmer climates. You can combat temperature-related weight gain by increasing your activity level, exercising more or reducing the amount of calories you consume. Keeping active will help increase your body's internal temperature and keep you warmer than inactivity.

Some people cannot tolerate exposure to cold. For example, people with Raynaud's syndrome cannot tolerate exposure to cold temperatures.[1] Cold temperature can cause their hands and feet to turn pale blue and feel painful. Reduce your chance of being exposed to cold by dressing in warm clothing. Wear protective gloves, shoes and outerwear. Don't expose yourself to cold water or air. Some people, such as hypothyroid patients, older people, vegans, thin people, etc. are less able to tolerate being exposed to cold temperatures than the average person. These people prefer and need to be warmly dressed because they are more likely to get sick from being exposed to cold temperatures.

Cold can affect people's emotions. Patients with depression often feel worse during winter. Seasonal Affective Disorder is a clinical condition that is caused by weather and a lack of sunlight.[2] Cold weather can cause emotional and physical discomfort and decrease your sense of joy in life. That is why cold climate regions are much less populated than warm climate regions. If you know that your depression gets worse or is triggered by cold weather or during winter, then you will be able to take proactive steps in order to successfully manage your depression.

Ice and snow in winter can increase your chance of being accidentally injured. More people slip and fall during cold weather than in summer. Also ice and snow increases car accidents. Driving during the first snow of the year or during severe snow storms can dramatically increase your risk of being in an accident. Reduce your outdoor activity during this kind of weather.

Exposure to Hot Temperatures and Your Health

Many people say that they feel their best if the outside temperature stays between 50 and 80 degrees Fahrenheit. That is ideal weather, but there are very few places in the world that have this kind of perfect and steady temperature. Most places are either too hot or too cold or are constantly changing from hot to cold or from sunny to cloudy. We have already discussed how cold temperatures can affect your health.

Now we can talk about how heat can affect your health. Different people have different tolerance levels to heat exposure. Some people say any temperature above 50 degrees Fahrenheit is too hot for them. Some people feel very comfortable in 90 degree weather. Your ability to tolerate warm and hot temperatures can depend on how you dress as well. You can get overheated, even in winter, if you wear too much clothing. Here are some common sense ways to reduce the effects of hot temperatures on your health.

Heat can affect your quality of sleep. Heat can stimulate your sympathetic nervous system which can cause you to sweat, make you feel excited and increase your mental activity. Some people describe this as feeling as though they can't "shut-off" their minds. Hot temperatures are very uncomfortable and can make it very difficult to fall or stay asleep.

Hot temperatures are not comfortable and may irritate your body and can cause you to become irritable, anxious or even depressed. Negative emotions can also contribute to poor sleep quality. Hot temperatures can affect your energy level and cause you to fatigue easily. Prepare emotionally for exposure to hot temperatures so you can reduce your chance of having a negative experience. When you feel irritable or negative emotions in hot weather and understand that you feel that way because of the weather, you will be better able to control yourself and not let your emotions create problems for yourself, your life, your family or friends.

Your risk of getting an intestinal tract infection will be greater during summer months. Infections of the gastrointestinal tract become more common in summer because food rots much faster in warmer temperatures and people tend to eat outdoors more frequently, thus causing foods to be kept at warmer temperatures for longer periods of time and not properly refrigerated. Because of these reasons, food poisoning cases dramatically increase during summer months.

Insects can contaminate your food, dining table and utensils with dysentery, cholera, rotavirus or other bacteria or viruses. Eating these foods can cause a digestive tract infection. People eat more raw vegetables and fruits during summer because there is a large variety in season. This can increase your chance of getting an intestinal infection as well. Take the time to wash raw foods well. Only eat foods that have been properly stored and heated or chilled to reduce your chance of getting a digestive tract infection. People can spread food-borne infections to each other by not properly washing their hands before preparing foods. Food-borne infection outbreaks occur in clusters because an infected supply of food is generally supplied regionally. To prevent this from happening to you, you need to be extra cautious in summer, especially if you travel to an area where a food-borne illness epidemic has broken out.[3]

Skin infections and damage are more common in hot temperatures. During hot weather people wear less clothing and get more sunburns, direct skin contact allergies, contact dermatitis, bug bites, scratches by plants or animals, etc. When you have an open wound on your skin your chance of getting infection will be higher, but you can dress properly to reduce your chance of skin infection. If you have diabetes or low immunity, a skin infection can cause big problems for you. Heat can cause skin pain, irritations or infections to worsen in severely obese people because heat can prevent sweat and skin secretions from being able to dry, thus causing bacteria to grow in folds of skin. So stay cool, dry and take good care of your skin during summer. Properly care for your infection to prevent it from getting worse.

Body infections increase in hot climates. Germs multiply and spread quicker in hot temperatures. Because of this, your chance of getting an infection will be much higher when you are in hotter climates. That is the main reason people who lived in southern regions closer to the equator during ancient times had shorter life spans than people in northern regions. Even today, infectious diseases are much more common in hotter climate regions. This is due to the increased number of mosquitoes and other disease-carrying insects that thrive in hot climates. Mosquitoes multiply heavily in summer and can spread malaria, dengue fever, yellow fever, etc.[4] Actively preventing mosquito and other insect bites can prevent you from being infected with these diseases.

Know your individual heat tolerance and reduce your risk of developing heat exhaustion or heatstroke. Everybody's tolerance to heat is different. Usually, people who have MS, hyperthyroid disease or are obese are more sensitive to heat because their bodies cannot adequately balance their internal temperature. Exposure to heat or warm temperatures can cause these people to feel uncomfortable very quickly. They may even panic or get sick when they feel hot. If you have one of these health conditions, you should try to reduce the amount of time you spend outdoors. You can prepare for being in hot weather by having an ice pack or body cooling system, cold water, a wide-brimmed hat, heat-reflective clothing, an umbrella and other items readily available and with you while you participate in outdoor activities or to cool your body when the weather is too hot for you.

It can be dangerous for you when the temperature outside is too hot (for example, above 90 degrees Fahrenheit) and your chance of getting heat exhaustion or heatstroke will be higher. You should drink plenty of water because water can produce sweat and prevent heatstroke. Reduce the amount of heavy physical work or exercise you do in extremely hot weather because heat can cause you to feel fatigued quickly. Also, your body produces heat when you're physically active and the heat added by the weather can increase your chance of getting heatstroke. Common symptoms of heatstroke include a lack of sweating (unless you have been exercising), nausea, vomiting, flushed skin, rapid breathing, rapid heartbeat, headache, muscle cramps, muscle weakness and confusion. In severe cases of heatstroke, you may lose consciousness. Heat exhaustion symptoms include heat cramps, headache, dizziness, lightheadedness, nausea and skin that is still perspiring. Heat exhaustion may be self-treated by drinking a cool beverage (non-alcoholic), immediately moving to an air-conditioned location or by taking a cool shower. Use your common sense when you experience any of these symptoms. Heatstroke requires immediate medical attention. Do not put your life in danger.[5]

If you are over 65 years old, you should use extra caution because your body's ability to tolerate heat reduces as you age. Your body's ability to feel the sensation of heat and balance its internal temperature also reduces as you age. These factors may cause you to be at a higher risk for getting heatstroke or seriously putting your life in danger before you are aware of it or even feel uncomfortable. If you have congestive heart failure or other serious ailments, such as kidney failure or COPD, you need to use extra caution because extreme heat can trigger heart attack, stroke or worsen your existing syndrome. If you already have had or are at high risk for having one of these diseases, then you should be extra cautious and do not put yourself at risk by being exposed to extremely hot temperatures.

Prevent dehydration. Because you sweat more in hot temperatures, it is easier for you to get dehydrated. You should drink more water to prevent becoming dehydrated because this can increase your chance of having heatstroke, kidney stone, heart attack, stroke, etc. Drink plenty of water to ensure that you have at least four to eight full bladders of urine a day.

Hot temperatures reduce your appetite. People want to eat less during summer months because extreme heat causes people to lose their appetites. Also, there are plenty of fresh fruits and vegetables available during summer, so people tend to eat fewer calories during summer months. People who live in warm and hot climates tend to eat fewer calories overall. This may cause nutritional deficiency. Although it is less common to eat high calorie foods such as meat, cheese, eggs, seafood, etc. during summer, if you have an existing nutritional deficiency, you should adjust your diet and increase your caloric intake in order to address these nutritional deficiencies. It is especially important to prevent nutritional deficiencies in children.

Humidity and Your Health

Rain can wash off pollution, dust and pollen from the air. It is good for your indoor environment to open the windows after it rains in order to get a fresh air exchange in your home or workplace. You can also go outside to exercise as a way to enjoy fresh air after it rains. Rain creates moisture in the air that is good for your respiratory system because your nose and windpipe function more effectively when the air is moistened. Moist air can reduce the burden your respiratory organs have to moisten air before it enters your lungs. Moist air is good for your skin because it can help prevent dry skin, skin dehydration and the appearance of skin wrinkles.

However, rain can affect your health negatively as well. When it is raining, atmospheric pressure lowers and can cause an increase in body aches. People who have RA, lupus, arthritis, headaches, or any type of pain syndrome or condition, body itching, psoriasis, surgical scars, etc. often feel more pain when it is raining or about to rain. Rain can increase people's chance of developing depression or worsen existing depression. Mentally preparing for rain can reduce the related fatigue and depression it can cause.

Moisture increases mold growth. Some people are allergic to mold and experience intensified symptoms during a rainy season or while in a damp, rainy area. If you have this problem, you can use a dehumidifier in your home to reduce the moisture in your home or you can move to a drier climate.

Prepare for Wind and Storm Conditions to Protect Your Health

Wind can blow away an inversion and reduce pollution in densely populated areas. Having cleaner air blown in to an area is good for the overall environment, especially in highly polluted areas, but wind can negatively affect your health when it stirs up dust, pollen and other allergens present in the air. This type of air is not healthy to breathe for people who have COPD, bronchitis, asthma, nasal allergies, etc. People who suffer from these types of respiratory conditions can feel their syndromes get worse during windy times. If you have these illnesses, you should probably stay indoors during windy weather conditions. If you must go outside when it is windy, you can wear a mask to reduce the chance of blowing dust affecting your health. It is best to reduce or avoid outdoor exercise during dusty or windy days as well.

When the wind is blowing it reduces your clothing's ability to protect (maintain) your body's temperature. Because of this, you will feel colder when the wind is blowing than when it is not blowing. When the wind is blowing, you can reduce your chance of developing body aches and pains and your risk of catching a cold by dressing in layers to protect yourself from wind. Reduce your outdoor activity on windy days, especially if you have an illness or if you don't feel good. You should prepare yourself for unexpected or severe temperature changes and dress properly for potential weather changes.

Strong winds created during tornados, hurricanes, storms, etc. can increase your chance of being involved in a wind-related accident. During extremely windy conditions, you can be blown over or hit by blowing debris. Wind can blow down trees and other materials and can cause serious injury or death. It is because of this that people who have experienced extreme wind storms often develop fear, stress and emotional damage (such as post-traumatic stress disorder). You can reduce your risk of experiencing extreme weather conditions by listening to weather reports and warnings. Be well-prepared in advance, stay indoors and avoid traveling during strong storms, unless it has been recommended that you evacuate. Stay in communication with your family and friends and have an emergency plan in place to reduce your risk of being harmed in an extreme storm.

The Effects of Living in a Dry Climate

Dry climates can affect your body's health because your upper respiratory system has to moistened air before it can enter your lungs. Dry air increases your nose, windpipe and lungs' burden; because of this, it is unhealthy for your respiratory system to constantly have to breathe in dry air. If you already have a respiratory disorder, dry air can worsen your syndrome. You can drink more water or use a humidifier to moisten your living and work environments as a way to reduce the effects of dry air on your health.

Dry air can also cause your skin to be drier and itchier. This is especially true for older people because their skin's secretion ability is reduced, but you can wear more clothes and apply natural oil on your skin to prevent your skin from the effects of dry air.

Chapter Eight

How to Break Up
with Your Cigarettes

In the past, over forty percent of adults in the United States[1] smoked cigarettes because they didn't know that smoking could cause serious health problems. Today, because of research and experience, there is a seemingly endless supply of information available about the medical and social costs of smoking. People often discuss the negative side effects that come with a smoking habit and there are even several different public organizations and private groups that are dedicated to educating young people to never start smoking and helping people, who already smoke, quit. You can find dozens of free sources online and through local community organizations to learn more about which quit smoking aids are available, usually at no or very low cost to you. As people have become more educated in America about smoking, the percentage of people who smoke has dropped. Unfortunately, over twenty percent of adults in the Unites States still smoke.[2]

Here are some of the health problems that can be caused by smoking.[3]

1. **Lung cancer** – Eighty percent of lung cancer patients are smokers.
2. **Throat cancer**
3. **Sinus cancer**
4. **Oral cancer**
5. **Asthma**
6. **COPD**
7. **Emphysema**
8. **Pneumonia**

Smoking lowers your respiratory system's ability to fight off and recover from injuries and illnesses. This increases your chance of developing any of the above health problems. Having a chronic lung disorder can make your life very difficult. Breathing may become extremely difficult and your illness may cause you to become disabled. Smoking can cause throat, sinus and oral cancers. Smoking can directly irritate your lungs, leading to COPD and emphysema. Chronic lung disorders can make completing necessary tasks in your day to day life much more difficult.

Smoking does not only damage your respiratory system; when you smoke, carcinogens and other toxins found in cigarettes can get into your blood stream.[4] The blood stream transports these poisons throughout your entire body and they can cause blood vessel damage and hardening of your veins. This is why smoking is known to cause or worsen osteoporosis and can contribute to your chances of having a heart attack or stroke. Smoking can also increase your risk of developing (in addition to those listed above) bladder, kidney, breast, colon, brain and other body organ cancers.[5]

So Why Do People Still Smoke?

Throughout my medical practice, I have discussed the subject of smoking with many smokers. I have asked them why they continue to engage in this unhealthy habit. The following is what I have learned about why people don't quit smoking.

Most smokers lack adequate health knowledge and education.
What I have discovered is that one of the main reasons people smoke is that they lack education or general knowledge about health. The less educated a person is, the more likely it is that they will smoke. The fact of the matter is that smoking can cause a variety of serious, painful health problems.

Most smokers lack motivation to quit. Most smokers do not have the motivation to quit because they currently do not see any immediate, negative effects caused by their smoking. So, they don't see any immediate reason to quit. Most people successfully quit smoking only after they have developed a health problem, such as having a stroke or heart attack, and their doctor has seriously recommended that they quit smoking.

Smoking cigarettes is an emotional and mental disorder. Smoking cigarettes can cause behavioral disorders. People who smoke may often use these disorders as reasons for not quitting. Some of these popular excuses include the following.

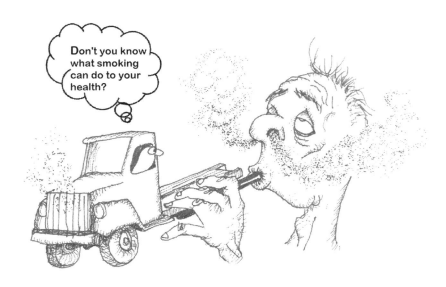

Many people use the notion that it is important to enjoy life as an excuse to justify smoking. They say that they just want to enjoy their time and that smoking is pleasurable. So, they continue to smoke. But, smoking can slowly deteriorate your quality of life and can shorten your life.

Some people use the excuse that smoking is an addiction. Because some people believe that smoking is an addiction and not a habit, they believe that it is simply too difficult or even impossible to quit. The effects caused by quitting smoking are more apparent in the changes of daily activities and behavior patterns of the person who quits rather than by actual physical withdrawal symptoms. Smokers experience few, if any, of the physical withdrawal symptoms that addictions cause. For example, if you are addicted to heroin, quitting can cause heart palpitations, restlessness, sleep disorders, muscle cramps, seizures and even death. But, when you quit cigarettes, none of these serious withdrawal symptoms occur. When quitting smoking, most of the withdrawal symptoms are emotional. People often report feeling anxious, stressed and mentally unable to relax.

Many people say that they have tried to quit, but nothing has worked for them. The truth is that these people are looking for an excuse or justification to keep their smoking habits, as opposed to actually looking for help. Although various methods can make it easier to quit, none of them can work unless you have truly committed yourself to kicking the habit.

Many people claim that they have been smoking for many years and feel fine. This is because people have varying tolerance levels to smoking. For example, if you have a respiratory disorder or asthma, your lung tolerance to smoking will be lower than a healthy person's tolerance. But, you cannot feel artery and lung inflammation that is caused by cigarette smoke until it causes more serious health problems. As you age, your body is not able to tolerate cigarette smoking as well as it can when you are younger. This is why that as smokers age, they develop more smoking-related health problems. There is no way to know how much smoking your body can tolerate before serious health problems begin to develop. It is best to quit smoking as soon as possible rather than taking a chance with your health.

Many people claim that they know a smoker who is healthy and has lived to an old age. This is a very common excuse among smokers who see no reason to quit smoking themselves. However, it is very likely that they do not know how much this person smoked, how deeply they inhaled, or other genetic, dietary and exercise factors that may have played a more significant role in this person's ability to live a long life.

Some people consider smoking to be a natural antidepressant. But, smoking can make you feel and look bad, which can worsen depression. Smoking may cause anxiety if you are concerned about how your smoking habit affects your children, family or friends. Concern for how your smoking influences how people think about you may cause you to feel stress and anxiety as well. You may even find yourself feeling uncomfortable around or avoiding friends and family members who disapprove of your smoking habit. The tension created between smokers and non-smokers in the same social group may even strain otherwise strong relationships. Smoking may affect how your workmates and employers view you and may add additional stress to your work environment. Additionally, smoking can make you anxious about your health.

Some people use smoking as an appetite suppressant. Over the years, I have had several of my patients tell me that they are worried that if they quit smoking, they will gain weight. They reason that being overweight will cause them as many or possibly more health problems than smoking, so they have decided to keep smoking and stay slim. Clearly, something that suppresses the appetite so drastically is not good for you. A habit that causes an artificially reduced appetite is not good for your digestive system. There are more efficient and healthy ways to lose weight or maintain your ideal weight that do not jeopardize your health.

Some people comfort themselves by bringing attention to the fact that they don't smoke as much as other people. This is another excuse that I hear quite frequently. People minimize the seriousness of their smoking habit by claiming that they only smoke a few cigarettes each day or that they only smoke socially, such as when they drink with their friends. But, smoking, regardless of how often you do it, reflects that you have weak willpower. Smoking cigarettes can damage your mental health by weakening self-control, self-discipline and willpower. If you continue to allow yourself to smoke, especially if you are young, this is not only a bad health habit, but also a bad mental habit.

Many people claim that it is okay for them to smoke because members of their family smoke. Smoking is not hereditary. Some people think that smoking must not be that bad when they see people working in the medical field, such as doctors and nurses, smoke. But, you need to remember that health professionals are human beings. They have the same weaknesses that can cause them to develop compulsive and damaging behaviors just like anyone else.

The majority of people who start smoking do so because of social pressure. The urge to fit in often causes people to make bad decisions, especially teenagers. It is common to discover that the majority of smokers began smoking as teenagers or very young adults. As we age, we are less likely to succumb to social pressures and, interestingly enough, the social pressures we experience as we age are influenced more by our desire to conform to healthy lifestyle choices and not the pressures of youth to rebel. Adults tend to associate with either smokers or non-smokers; therefore, it is highly unlikely that established adults will take-up smoking later in life.

Stubbornness can prevent some people from being able to quit smoking. One of my patients, who had late-stage lung cancer, was still smoking. I asked her why she was still smoking and she told me that even though she had lung cancer, she did not believe that it had been caused by smoking. She went on to say, "The lord loves us, and the lord made tobacco. So how can tobacco be hurtful?" (She died shortly after that.) But, we can extend this logic and see that it is not rational at all. Nature is full of examples of plants and animals that are not safe for us. Poison ivy can cause great discomfort; as can interacting with grizzly bears and sharks. Environmental elements do not solely exist for human use.

Reasons That May Create a Desire for You to Quit Smoking

Love for your family. A patient of mine had tried to quit smoking multiple times and his family had been begging him to quit for years. One day his four year old granddaughter visited him and asked, "Grandpa, do you love me or smoking more?" He answered, "I love you more, sweetie." The granddaughter responded, "Well, grandpa, the smoke stinks and it hurts my nose. Can you stop it?" He was very surprised to hear her say that. But, because he loved her so much he put his cigarette out and never smoked again.

Need to meet religious and social expectations. People who grow up in religious or socially involved households tend to not pick up smoking during their youth. People may tend to avoid smoking in order to fit into certain social circles or to appease a mate. Giving up smoking for the comfort of your friends and family is not unreasonable. You may find encouragement to quit smoking from these very social circles. You most likely will find that many of your friends and family members are more than willing to do whatever they can to help you quit smoking.

Health issues may encourage people to stop smoking. People, who are otherwise healthy but develop high blood pressure or breathing problems, may quit smoking quickly in an attempt to protect their already damaged health. Some people develop smoking related disorders (such as COPD) and get to the point where the need to carry an oxygen tank around with them. Unfortunately, even at this point, some people cannot quit, so they continue to smoke. A patient of mine found herself in this situation. It was only after becoming disabled from two heart attacks and three strokes that she was finally able to quit smoking.

You can always find an excuse to not quit smoking. But, if you become aware and try to remain aware of the fact that smoking habits are behavioral disorders more than anything else; this new perspective can make it easier for you to quit. It may help you to think about those around you and your loved ones. Smoking may reduce your life span and the time you have with your loved ones. Remember that smoking around others jeopardizes their health as well as your own. I have known people who have put their children on allergy medications because they could not stop smoking even though their children were desperately allergic to the second-hand smoke being created in their homes. How irresponsible it is for parents, or for any of us, to risk the health of those we love, live with and work with because we cannot or will not break a habit.

Smoking can create a huge financial burden for you, your family and society. Unfortunately, the majority of people who smoke have fairly low incomes.[6] Smoking reflects a poor knowledge of financial management and investments. Cigarettes and other tobacco products are expensive and heavily taxed. Sooner or later, you will have medical costs related to smoking.

Second-hand smoke can make your family members ill, thus increasing the cost of their medical care. Additionally, smoking around young children can teach them that it is okay to smoke and may lead them to develop poor habits as they grow up. Or, as I mentioned earlier, can cause them to develop allergies or other health problems that create a financial burden for your family as well.

Some people try to quit smoking but have a very difficult time doing so because they do not go about the process properly. In my practice, I have helped hundreds of people quit smoking and remain quitters on their own without additional assistance from me or stop smoking products.

A Few Tips That May Improve Your Long-term Success of Kicking the Habit

Quit smoking cold turkey. People who try to quit smoking by slowly cutting down how many times they smoke during the day actually end up enjoying cigarettes more than they did before. This makes it more difficult to quit.

Don't be afraid of the detoxifying process when you quit smoking. As your lungs begin to clear after the first few weeks of not smoking, you may find that you are coughing a lot. Some people are very concerned that if they quit smoking they will cough too much. Don't be afraid if this occurs. It only takes two or three weeks for your lungs to finish cleansing themselves. Drinking a stop smoking tea or other lung immunity building tea may help you get through this cleansing process. You may find that drinking tea will become an enjoyable and healthy new habit for you.

Do not overeat. Smoking suppresses the appetite and makes food less tasty. So, after you quit smoking, you will probably enjoy eating more and may have a larger appetite. It is important that you combat the urge to eat more after you quit smoking. Be aware of what foods you are eating. Chew slowly and enjoy the process of tasting and eating healthy foods.

Do not allow yourself to eat more sugar after you quit smoking. Many people develop serious food cravings, mostly sugar cravings, when going through process of quitting smoking. Eating more sugar can cause weight gain. A patient of mine gained sixty pounds the first year after she quit smoking because every time she craved a cigarette she would resist the urge by eating candy. Again, try drinking herbal teas or other beverages that are unsweetened. (Avoid artificial sweeteners, as they can lead to health problems.) Or, go for a walk or engage in a distracting activity if you think that you feel hungry or bored.

Stay busy and pick up new hobbies to help you quit. If you are in the habit of smoking after a meal or during work breaks, try going for a short walk or do some other type of activity during these times to help you change your habits and keep your mind occupied.

Build a support system to help you quit smoking. Quit with a loved one, family member, a friend or join a support group. Quitting with support from someone else gives both of you the perseverance and dedication needed to successfully quit.

Educate yourself about the negative health effects caused by smoking. When you crave a cigarette, find and study information about the health benefits of quitting cigarettes. Have articles from news sources, health sites, research reports, etc. readily available so that you can review them frequently and remind yourself how much you are improving your health and quality of life by quitting.

Replace your smoking habit with positive, healthy habit. Exercise, meditate or find another activity to occupy your mind and time. Do not smoke out of boredom or to relieve tension. Avoid social situations that encourage you to smoke.

After you have stopped smoking you may still remember the habit fondly, even years later. But, if you smoke again, you will probably not enjoy it and it will take a while for you to find it pleasurable again. Keep your resolve to living a healthier, smoke-free life. Do not let yourself relapse.

Chapter Nine

Overcoming Addictions
Taking Back Control of Your Life

Alcohol Abuse

For thousands of years, people all over the world have been drinking and enjoying alcoholic beverages for pleasure. Before anesthesia became common, alcohol was used as a pain killer for surgeries and other medical procedures. Nowadays, alcohol is affordable, so most people can easily access it. In some cultures, the majority of the population's daily activities include drinking alcoholic beverages. In some countries, alcohol is consumed in place of water at meals because alcohol is easier and cheaper to access than clean water. Drinking alcohol can often lead to serious health problems and alcoholism. Because of this, it is best to avoid drinking alcohol as part of your daily lifestyle or habit.

It is commonly known that drinking too much alcohol can lead to all sorts of physical and emotional health problems as well as legal and social problems. Here is a brief list of some of the negative effects commonly associated with drinking too much alcohol.

Drunk Driving –approximately 10,000 people in the United States were killed in alcohol related driving accidents in 2010 and thousands more were injured.[1] Almost one and a half million people get arrested for drunk driving in the United States each year.[2] Drunk driving kills people, burdens the legal system, uses already scarce resources of law enforcement, increases financial burdens, increases insurance costs, etc.[3]

Arteriosclerosis –a hardening and loss of elasticity of the arteries can develop throughout your entire body including in arteries of major organs such as the heart, kidneys and lungs. This disease, although not uncommon as we age, develops with acceleration when you consume too much alcohol and can lead to greater health issues due to restricted blood flow such as blood clot, stroke, heart attack, permanent heart damage, aseptic necrosis of the head of the femur (leading to the need for a hip replacement), etc.

Liver Damage –alcohol is processed in your body through your liver. After alcohol is processed (metabolized), ethyl aldehyde, a chemical yielded from the process of breaking down alcohol, can damage your liver, cause alcohol induced hepatitis, fatty liver and lead to cirrhosis (liver failure). Alcohol induced cirrhosis is the one of the leading causes of liver cirrhosis in America.[4]

Pancreas Damage –alcohol abuse can cause you to develop pancreatitis. Pancreatitis is inflammation of the pancreas and can cause upper abdominal pain, back pain, hydroperitoneum (water retention in the abdomen), nausea, vomiting and internal bleeding. It often becomes a chronic condition in people who drink too much alcohol. Pancreatitis may also lead to the onset of Type I Diabetes or pancreatic cancer.

Brain Damage –alcohol abuse can cause permanent memory loss and short-term memory loss. Long-term alcohol abuse can cause the early onset of dementia.

Nerve Disorders –alcohol abuse can lead to sleep disorders, numbness in the hands and feet (neuropathy), rapid heartbeat, elevated blood pressure, migraines and other conditions that are caused by alcohol's damaging effects on the nervous system.

Increased Risk of Metabolic Syndrome –metabolic syndrome is a combination of diseases that includes high cholesterol, high blood pressure, elevated blood sugar and a high percentage of abdominal fat. This syndrome can lead to diabetes, cardiovascular disease, heart attack, stroke or cancer. If you already have metabolic syndrome, then drinking alcohol will most likely worsen your syndrome.

Digestive System Damage –alcohol abuse, especially when it leads to nausea and vomiting, can cause severe digestive disorders including gastritis, irritable bowel syndrome, chronic heartburn, intestinal diseases, cancer, etc. Alcohol, especially beer, increases the amount of calories you consume. This can cause you to gain weight or develop a "beer belly" which places additional stress on your digestive system and your entire body.

Emotional Problems and Disorders –alcohol can make people more talkative and cause them to feel and express their emotions to a stronger degree. For example, the effects of alcohol may cause an otherwise quiet and happy person to express extreme sadness, anger, etc. Or, it may cause a normally unhappy person feel extremely happy and outgoing. Alcohol affects your ability to make good choices and can cause you to engage in unprotected sex which can lead to sexually transmitted infections and unwanted pregnancies. Poor judgment increases your chance of being involved in a serious physical accident because alcohol reduces your ability to pay attention, reaction time and vision.

Alcohol abuse can cause depression and stress. It may contribute to a person's loss of motivation to take care of oneself, to study and complete their educational assignments, to work or hold a job or obey the law. Alcohol abuse can stress and damage personal relationships with family, friends and workmates. Additionally, alcoholism negatively affects children in a multitude of ways including disappointment, loss of closeness to the alcoholic parent and, potentially, the development of similar negative drinking habits.

Drug Use –it is not uncommon for alcohol abuse to lead to drug use and abuse in many different forms from using marijuana or harder drugs to developing an addiction to prescription drugs. Alcohol, when mixed with certain prescription drugs, can be deadly. You should pay attention to warnings that advise you to avoid alcohol if you are taking prescription medication.

Birth Defects –Fetal Alcohol Syndrome is a serious disorder that can cause severe mental and physical deformities.[5] Alcohol abuse can cause many other types of birth defects and prevents a child from having their best possible start in life when they are born with so many existing health issues. The burden for them and society is astronomical.[6]

Reasons People Drink Alcohol

There are a multitude of reasons why people drink alcohol. There are some widely held misconceptions about alcohol that people often use to justify their drinking habits. The following is a list of some common reasons people drink alcohol and some examples of common misconceptions about alcohol.

Misconception 1: Red Wine is Beneficial for Health –it is

commonly believed that red wine contains antioxidants that can slow down the aging process. If you do an internet search related to "red wine antioxidants" you will find many articles claiming that red wine is actually very healthy. Therefore, many people try to drink a glass of red wine daily or multiple times a week in order to slow down the aging process. You may hear of different medical doctors who recommend adding red wine to the diet as a way to maintain good health. However, there are a couple of reasons why you should question the assertion that red wine is good for you. First of all, I think that there are much healthier antioxidant sources than red wine. Second, many people economically benefit from promoting red wine as being "healthy". Also, alcohol, including wine, only tastes good after you have developed a taste for it. So, the more you drink, the tastier it gets; and the tastier it gets, the more you will buy. This can easily lead to alcohol abuse. No matter how beneficial the antioxidants in wine may be, the alcohol that wine contains is no less toxic than any other type of alcoholic beverage.

Misconception 2: Alcohol Relieves Stress –some people think that

alcohol is a natural antidepressant and sleep aid. Occasionally drinking alcohol can be beneficial to help you fall asleep if acute stress (short-lived, related to a specific event) causes you to not be able to fall asleep. But alcohol can also excite your brain which can end up making it more difficult for you to fall asleep. Regularly drinking alcohol as a way to fall asleep can cause you to develop a sleep disorder in the long run. If you drink to help yourself fall asleep, do so only occasionally. Don't make it a habit that you have to have a drink in order to fall asleep. Drinking alcohol regularly to address a sleep problem may worsen your existing sleep disorder and may even lead to other health problems.

Misconception 3: Alcohol Reduces Pain –it is true that alcohol can

act as a natural pain reliever. Drinking enough of it can actually cause you to pass out. That is why, in the past, alcohol was used as a narcotic and for anesthesia purposes. Alcohol can help temporarily relieve your entire body's pain and conditions such as arthritis and fibromyalgia. But, surely, you should not drink alcohol daily for pain relief because the pain relief that comes from drinking alcohol is short-lived and, in most cases, will cause additional health problems and may increase your level of pain over time. If you have gout, drinking alcohol can worsen your condition. If you drink too much at once, you may experience a hangover or digestive problems that most likely will immediately cause your other existing pain conditions to feel worse as well.

Misconception 4: Alcohol Relieves Emotional Distress –alcohol is almost like a natural antidepressant; it makes you excited, happy, relaxed and talkative. This is the main reason why alcohol is so widely used. But, it is important to remember that alcohol is toxic. Drinking too much of it can cause you to pass out, black out and, in extreme cases, can cause death. Regular alcohol abuse can lead to depression and severe emotional disorders. The physical and social damage caused by a drinking problem can cause you to develop depression, especially if your drinking problem causes you to have legal problems, lose your job or to be separated from your family.

Misconception 5: Beer Helps with Milk Production –although this is, in part, true, drinking beer also has negative side effects, such as weight gain and a small amount of alcohol will be present in the produced milk. Eating barley or using hops in an herbal tea are much healthier ways to increase milk production.

All of the above examples are some commonly held ideas about how alcohol can be beneficial. But, regardless of the potential health benefits of alcohol, drinking too much too often will eventually worsen preexisting problems and most likely cause new ones. Many people know that alcohol abuse causes health problems, but millions of people continue to drink alcohol regularly.

Excuses People Use as Reasons to Keep Drinking Alcohol

Excuse 1: Alcohol Relieves Emotional Pain –people use alcohol to numb the pain of a bad childhood, bad memories, loss of a loved one, severe depression, post-war trauma, post-traumatic stress or a negative home life. Many people are not consciously aware of the fact that they are using alcohol to numb their emotional pain. Fortunately, there are much better ways to manage depression. Other approaches may take longer to achieve the result of feeling better, but in the long run, will be more beneficial for your mind and body. If you are struggling with sadness, lack of motivation, depression, feeling misguided or other emotional issues that are taking away from your quality of life, it is best to talk to a professional counselor or therapist instead of self-medicating. Ask for help from family and friends. There are always ays to get the help you need without harming yourself or the ones you love.

Excuse 2: *Teenage Drinking is a Normal Rebellion* –this is the most popular excuse for adolescents and young adults. Although teenage drinking causes much pain for loved ones, especially parents and siblings, it really does the most damage to the drinker. Some parents may not take teenage drinking seriously because they engaged in it themselves when they were young and may believe that it is a rite of passage. Teenage drinking should not be tolerated and should be addressed immediately to prevent long-term damage to the child's physical, emotional and financial future well-being.

Excuse 3: *Drinking is Part of the Culture* –for example, in Chinese culture a popular saying is, "If you do not have an alcoholic beverage with dinner, then it is not a real dinner." Additionally, some people drink because of the social circumstances, such as attending a party or being invited to a meal, because it is regarded as insulting to their host if they do not drink alcohol when offered.

Excuse 4: *Alcohol is Addictive* –drinking regularly, even it if it just one glass of wine or one beer a day, can cause you to develop an alcohol addiction. Alcohol addictions range in levels of severity. Some people may be addicted to alcohol but never display signs of being drunk or may not drink to the level of becoming visibly drunk. But they are still addicted to alcohol, because if they are withheld from drinking alcohol, they will develop withdrawal symptoms similar to someone who is recovering from being drunk. Some of these withdrawal symptoms may include poor balance, confusion, rapid heartbeat, headache, vomiting and, in severe cases, hallucinations. It is your choice to claim addiction as an excuse for drinking alcohol. There are many programs and ways of getting help to break alcohol addiction, but no one can help you until you make the decision to quit. When you do decide to quit, reach out for help; someone will be there to help you.

Excuse 5: *Alcoholism is Genetic* –many people claim that alcoholism runs in their family. They claim that since they are genetically prone to alcoholism, they can't control their actions. However, I believe that alcoholism is not a disease that must manifest itself. Your family's mental health history and the habits of your close relatives are far more responsible for what is called a genetic disposition to alcoholism. Just because you may be predisposed to develop alcoholism doesn't mean that you have to develop alcoholism. Knowing your genetic factors should help you to reduce your risk of becoming alcoholic because you can proactively make choices not to drink alcohol and avoid environments that influence your ability to abstain from using alcohol. You may not be able to change your genetics, but you can control yourself and choose to never become alcoholic.

Excuse 6: Alcoholism is a Disease –it is very easy to dismiss responsibility for yourself when a doctor tells you that alcoholism is a disease. But, the truth is that alcoholism is the result of bad habits. Don't let the label of "alcoholism is a disease" become a crutch for you to not take responsibility for your health and well-being. You can choose to stop drinking and continue to choose not to drink every day after that.

Excuse 7: Drinking Alcohol is a Good Way to Enjoy Life – although alcohol has widely been used for entertainment throughout history, there are far better and healthier ways to enjoy life. How tragic it is when our desire to enjoy life leads us to developing serious health problems, harming others or creating legal and financial troubles for ourselves and possibly our families. The side effects of drinking alcohol will diminish the quality of your life and may actually prevent you from being able to enjoy the rest of your life. Use common sense when making entertainment decisions. Your social life should not revolve around alcohol.

Some Examples of the Hardships That Alcohol Abuse Can Cause

Alcohol is one of the Main Reasons for Family Problems –including domestic problems between wives and husbands and parents and children. Alcohol abuse can lead you to neglect your loved ones, especially your children and yourself. If you do not take responsibility for yourself, how can you live up to your obligation to take care of your family? Children who grow up without the attention or love of an alcoholic parent usually develop severe emotional disorders. Do not allow yourself to be responsible for the long-term and severe damage of your own child.

Many Alcoholics Have Shortened Lifespans –when young people drink excessively, they can cause severe physical damage that can cause them to die young. Having a parent outlive their alcoholic child is extremely painful. Leaving behind a mate or young children who no longer have one of their parents to love and care for them are

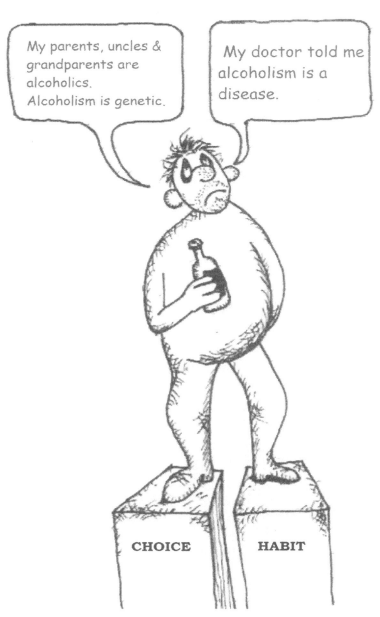

**Stop looking for excuses.
Accept personal responsibility for your addictions.**

extremely painful and devastating experiences. You can avoid this by loving your family enough to take care of yourself and control your alcohol use.

Loss of Personal Relationships –family and friends often drift away from those who develop alcohol issues. Sometimes families have to leave an alcoholic member to protect themselves from violence and financial danger. The feeling of abandonment and loneliness can lead to severe depression and can trigger suicidal thoughts.[7]

Physical and Emotional Damage –it is difficult to treat alcohol induced health damage, even after you have quit drinking. I know many people who continue to endure the negative effects of alcoholism for years after having quit drinking. I have treated several patients who have spent years suffering from the effects of their drinking. One of my patients developed pancreatitis and Type I Diabetes because of his alcohol abuse. Even though he hasn't had a drink in twenty years, he will have diabetes for the rest of his life because diabetes that is caused by physical damage to the pancreas cannot be treated with diet and exercise. One of my older patients was experiencing the burden of having to care full-time for her fifty year old daughter who had developed severe dementia and could no longer care for herself because of her alcohol abuse. One of my female patients was also fifty years old and had been struggling with alcohol abuse for decades. She wasn't able to work because she lived in constant pain because her alcoholism had damaged her hip joint so severely that she couldn't stand. (Aseptic necrosis of the femur head is a common cause of necessary hip replacement surgeries for people who have abused alcohol.[8]) She wasn't eligible to receive a surgical replacement because she couldn't stop drinking long enough to be able to undergo anesthesia. After thirty-five years of alcohol abuse (drinking six beers a day) a patient of mine is waiting for a liver transplant because he developed severe liver cirrhosis, which has also caused him to experience a lack of appetite, nutritional deficiency, kidney inflammation, fatigue, edema, bloating and anemia.

Injury or Death of Yourself and Others –again, every year over 10,000 people in the United States die as a result of someone drinking and driving. As mentioned earlier, the health damages caused by drinking alcohol can greatly shorten the length of your life. You can injure yourself or others when you participate in activities while your focus, vision and balance are reduced. When alcohol impairs your ability to make good judgments, you may engage in dangerous, life-threatening activities that include reckless driving, work-related accidents, extreme sports or tricks, taking other risks or physical challenges or engaging in high-risk sexual activities.

People Lose Respect for You –it can be humiliating to get extremely drunk, vomit and pass out; or to be at a social event and behavior in a manner outside of generally accepted social norms. This type of behavior may cause you to lose your job, your status in the community or your friends. Most people lose respect for their family and friends when they experience them acting out in a drunken state.

Hopefully, this information has changed your awareness of the true effects of drinking alcohol, and will help you to change your drinking habits or quit drinking altogether in order to prevent health problems. The most important thing to acknowledge when attempting to quit or cut down your alcohol intake is to realize the seriousness of the health and emotional problems that drinking too much alcohol causes.

How to Quit Drinking and Prevent Alcoholism

It is important for you to be able to take an honest look at yourself and know what type of personality you have. This will help you make decisions that will most effectively help you quit drinking. From my experience, I have found that most people fit into four different personality types when it comes to their ability to stop drinking.

1. *People with strong willpower or an easily moldable personality.* Some people are able to remain totally steadfast in their attempt to quit drinking because they are the types of people who, after committing themselves to something, are able to stick to it. These types of people usually do not find it too difficult to quit. Some people are easily influenced by others and are able to stop drinking when convinced it is the best choice for them to make.

2. *Those that need constant pressure.* Some people need constant pressure and support from their spouse, loved ones, religious beliefs, support group (such as Alcoholics Anonymous), etc. to keep making the right decisions on a daily basis. If you are this type of person, you need to find a positive source of constant pressure to help you quit and prevent relapse.

3. *Some people need to experience the negative effects of drinking in order to have the motivation to quit.* Often times, these people experience serious health problems before taking the need to quit drinking seriously. Unfortunately, these kinds of people tend to quit when it is already too late.

4. *People who need physical intervention.* Some people need to be forcefully or physically cut off from alcohol by having all access to alcohol taken away from them or by being placed in a controlled environment where they are not able to access alcohol. Some people willingly go to treatment centers while others are forced into treatment or jail because of the effects caused by their inability to control their alcohol intake.

If you drink, be moderate. Do not drink daily. Drinking occasionally – and not to the point of getting drunk –should not have too much of an effect on your health. Drinking too often can easily lead to alcoholism.

Drinking infrequently, but getting drunk every time you drink (binge drinking), is very bad for your health. These types of drinkers tend to have enough willpower to quit, so once they realize how unhealthy drinking to the point of getting drunk is, they can usually cut down their drinking or abstain from it altogether.

If you have previously experienced an alcohol-related social problem such as having been arrested, having caused an accident or having instigated a violent act; or if you have had an alcohol-related health problem such as alcoholism, digestive disorders, hepatitis, pancreatitis etc., then you should avoid drinking altogether.

If your personality matches one of the personalities outlined above in 2-4, then you need to continuously educate yourself about the negative effects of alcohol, seek the right kind of professional help and, most of all, take responsibility for yourself and pursue the treatment that will most effectively help you quit.

If you get drunk regularly, stopping cold turkey can lead to withdrawal syndrome (severe alcohol cravings, anxiety, heart palpitations, sweating, shivering, poor balance and hallucinations). In these cases, it is necessary to get professional help that will allow you to slowly cut down alcohol intake. If you experience withdrawal syndrome, it is important to go to a doctor and make sure your physical condition is closely monitored. In some cases severe withdrawal syndrome can cause severe health problems including triggering seizures or heart attacks.

Once you realize that drinking will eventually lead to severe and unpleasant health problems, it becomes much easier to quit. Keep reminding yourself of the facts and do as much research as possible in order to sustain the willpower you need to cut down how much you drink or to help you quit drinking altogether.

Illicit and Prescription Drug Abuse and Misuse

Drug abuse and addiction includes the improper use of both illegal and legal drugs. Some legal drugs, such as most narcotic pain medications, are made from the same ingredients that illegal drugs are made from – opium. Other popularly abused drugs include marijuana, cocaine, heroin and methamphetamines. All of these drugs can lead to varying levels of abuse and addiction in people. The most popularly misused and heavily addictive drugs are opium products such as heroin and narcotic pain medications. Opiate derived prescription medications can have the same negative effects as heroin. Whether used illegally or legally, these drugs can seriously affect your health and quality of life.[9]

For purposes of providing an example, I will discuss only the effects of opiates because I have found in my experience that they are the most widely misused drugs. Overall, I have found in my practice in the United States for the last fifteen years that an average of one in four of all of my patients regularly take some form of a narcotic drug. Most of the effects of opiates can be applied to the misuse of other drugs as well. Common health ailments that I have associated with the overuse of narcotics include the following.

Digestive Disorders –opiates in your body can cause nausea, vomiting, liver damage, constipation and other digestive problems. If you have hepatitis or liver problems, then ingesting opiates will worsen your preexisting problems.

Sleep Disorders –opiates can cause drowsiness and chronic sleep disorders. The opiate high can make it difficult to fall asleep for days at a time. Long-term drug abuse can cause severe sleep disorders. Many doctors treat this problem by prescribing sleeping pills, which is why many people who take narcotics also take sleeping pills.

Attention Disorders –when you are high on opiates, your ability to pay attention is greatly diminished, which can cause you to be involved in an auto or other type of accident. This is why professional drivers, such as pilots and truck drivers, and those who operate heavy machinery are not allowed to be on opiates while on the job. Although the law does not prohibit regular citizens from driving while on these drugs, doing so puts yourself and others in danger. Long-term use of these drugs can cause permanent attention disorders (that can affect your ability to focus long after you have quit using narcotics), which also increases your chances of getting into a car or work-related accident.

Permanent Brain Damage –overdosing on opiates increases your chances of having a stroke and can lead to paralysis. Even just short-term drug abuse can cause lasting attention disorders, make it difficult to focus and can cause permanent memory loss. Long-term drug abuse can cause severe attention disorders and dementia. This is why some of my older, less energetic patients who take pain medication on a regular basis seem like they have dementia. While on these drugs or medications the brain is used less, which slowly diminishes the brain's abilities and functioning capabilities, and increases the chances of developing dementia.

Lack of Motivation –loss of motivation to take care of yourself, your family, your career and other personal relationships is a socially damaging side effect of drug abuse. This is commonly referred to as failure to thrive and is especially harmful to people over age fifty-five that have drug or alcohol addictions.[10] Drug abuse almost always causes emotional and financial problems for families. Without motivation to develop relationships with family members, people lack the joy and support that comes from being part of a healthy family unit. Your loss of interest in living may lead you to developing other emotional problems or disorders such as anxiety and depression.

A drug addiction increases your chances of engaging in criminal behavior. When addicted to drugs some people (especially younger adults) will do anything to get them. These people's total focus in life becomes getting their next high. Their addiction causes them to lose interest in everything else and they are willing to risk anything to get their next drug fix. Lack of concern for personal well-being and life can cause people to engage in high-risk activities such as unprotected sex or sharing needles; both of these can lead to serious, life-threatening diseases.

Other Side Effects –opiates can affect your ability to maintain your physical balance which increases the chance of falling and other injuries. Opiate use can decrease your alertness and cause dizziness, which is particularly dangerous for older people. These drugs can trigger and worsen serious health conditions. Drug abuse can trigger asthma or COPD attacks, cause heart problems, seriously worsen liver, prostate and urinary conditions and negatively affect your sexual health.

A drug-induced high can cause people to experience extreme hallucinations that can prompt dangerous reactions. There are plenty of tragic and disturbing reports of violent crimes that occur when people are in drug-induced, altered mental states.

Drug overdose can cost you your life. It has been estimated that over 50,000 deaths are caused by unintentional drug overdose or misuse (including prescription and illegal drugs) in the United States each year.[11] The effects of misusing drugs impact your health and your life and can be irreversible. Tragically, the rate of drug abuse in this country is increasing.

How to Quit a Drug Addiction

Quitting drugs is similar to quitting alcohol. You need motivation to quit using drugs. You can use the approaches to quit alcohol described above to quit using drugs as well. You have to be devoted to quitting before you can make any progress. Quitting drugs is just as difficult as quitting drinking, but the withdrawal syndrome caused from quitting some drugs can actually be more severe than alcohol withdrawal syndrome. Withdrawal syndrome from heroin can include severe restlessness, anxiety, insomnia, extremely rapid heartbeat, elevated blood pressure, body aches and pain and may even trigger seizures or cause death. The more intense and long-term your drug use is, the harder it will be to quit. Most people may find that they have to go off drugs slowly and cannot quit cold turkey. This includes both illegal drugs and addictions to prescription medications, especially opiate-based painkillers. Although severe withdrawal syndrome should not last for more than one or two weeks, it is extremely important for a person going through the withdrawal process to be medically monitored and receive the appropriate professional assistance they need.

Widespread alcohol and drug use or addiction can deteriorate a citizen's performance in society. This reduction in productivity can devastate not only the economic stability of the individual or family, but can diminish the community or nation as a whole.[12, 13, 14] For example, in the early 1800's opium became widely used in China. The country went from being economically sound to experiencing a serious economic crash. The rampant opiate drug use caused a downfall of the nation as a whole. It is easy to blame the government for economic woes, but the personal habits of a country's citizens has a lot more to do with the well-being of a nation's economy than most people realize. For the betterment of the nation as a whole, we should make an effort to stop alcohol and drug abuse.

Chapter Ten

Reduce Your Risk of Being Involved in an Automobile Accident

We usually refer to automobile crashes as accidents, but what is an accident? An accident is an event that takes place without expectation, in an instant and happens by chance.[1] If, for example, a car crash happens because a driver has a heart attack while driving, then the car crash is indeed an accident. But most vehicle crashes are the result of preventable, dangerous circumstances, like when a driver does not pay attention or is under the influence of alcohol, illegal drugs or prescription medications. A friend of mine who is a police officer told me that throughout his twenty years of service less than one percent of car crashes he examined were caused by real accidents (such as heart attack , seizure, automobile malfunction, etc.).

Nowadays, vehicles have become the main mode of transportation. We use them to go to work, shopping, school, travel, etc. Most people actually enjoy driving their own car and prefer it to public transportation. Like everything in life, there are both good and bad things about driving. Having your own vehicle to drive may be convenient, but driving in a car is risky. Light passenger vehicles (personal cars, trucks, SUVs, etc.) are the deadliest modes of transportation.[2] According to the U.S. census bureau in 2011, over 33,000 people died from car accidents in the United States.[3]

Most people who use a car as their main type of transportation will be involved in one or more car accidents in their lifetime. Thousands of people suffer moderate to severe injuries caused by car accidents each year. Common injuries include neck injuries such as whiplash, bone fractures, soft tissue sprains or tears, broken bones, cuts and lacerations, brain injuries, blindness, spinal injuries, disabilities, post-traumatic stress disorder, emotional trauma, and even severe financial hardship caused by repair and replacement expenses, medical expenses, increased insurance rates, lost wages, etc. The stress and worry of the financial hardships related to auto accidents can cause emotional and post-traumatic symptoms to worsen. Motor vehicle crashes are the leading cause of death among those aged five to thirty-four years old in the U.S. More than 2.3 million adult drivers and passengers were treated in emergency departments as the result of being injured in motor vehicle crashes in 2009. The economic impact is also notable – the lifetime cost of crash-related deaths and injuries among drivers and passengers was $70 billion in 2005 alone.[4]

Can vehicle accidents be avoided? No, not entirely. However, a majority of accidents can be avoided if you prepare yourself and drive more carefully. Here are some factors that may reduce your risk of being involved in a car crash.

Speed –speeding is one of the main causes of vehicle crashes. Approximately one-third of vehicle crashes are caused by speeding. Speeding involves driving faster than conditions permit, not just driving over the posted speed limit. Posted speed limits are set with much consideration. Concerned and responsible citizens will respect and follow speed limit laws. Driving over the speed limit can place your own life and the life of others in serious danger.[5]

Ways to Slow Down

1. Provide yourself with enough time to get to your destination without rushing.
2. Inattentiveness and distractions can cause unconscious speeding. Focus one hundred percent of your attention on driving. Don't

daydream, play with radio or temperature controls, eat, reach for items in the backseat or attend to passengers while you are driving.

3. Do not ever drive under the influence of new medications (that you haven't had time to discover what your potential reaction to them is), alcohol or drugs. All of these things may cause you to lose your ability to control your driving speed.

4. Bad driving habits, like competitive and aggressive driving, can cause you to get into the habit of speeding.

5. Intentionally adjust your speed for weather conditions, road hazards, traffic patterns, on other conditions that require you to pay more attention to your driving environment. Reduce your speed for rain, fog, below freezing temperatures, snow, icy roads, heavy bumper-to-bumper traffic, road work, road blocks, etc. Remember that the speed limit is set as the maximum acceptable speed for clear and optimal weather conditions.

6. Driving too slow for the flow of traffic can increase your chances of having vehicle crash as well, especially in heavily trafficked areas and cities. If you are driving slowly down a freeway or densely populated roadway, you place yourself in dangers and others in danger from coming up behind you too quickly or trying to pass you. You become a hazard when you block the flow of traffic with excessively slow speeds. This is true for people who pull trailers and other items behind them as well.

Distracted Driving – The Leading Cause of Automobile Accidents

When cars are moving very fast accidents can happen in the blink of an eye. In one moment, your life can change dramatically. If you are involved in a vehicle crash, it is very likely that you will suffer from some type of pain and injury. You may be facing astronomical bills after an accident, even if you have good insurance. You may have to pay heavy fines or even spend time in jail if you are legally held responsible for the accident. You may even have to spend the rest of your life carrying the guilt (emotional distress) of having injured another person.

Most people do not drive with their full attention. They are doing other things while driving such as texting, eating, reading, looking at a video or navigation system, talking on their cellphone, etc. Or, they are driving under the influence of anger, alcohol, drugs or medicine. They may be daydreaming or distracted their surroundings or passengers, etc. (Sadly, some of these events are not counted in distracted driving activity statistics.) Distracted driving is dangerous and can be deadly; eighteen percent of all injury crashes were caused by distracted driving in 2010.[6]

Ways to Reduce Distraction

Understand the true dangers involved in driving including excessive speeds, drinking alcohol and driving while distracted. Most people, especially teenagers and young adults, frequently drive with only one hand or even use their leg to steer, so they can put on makeup, talk on the phone, text, interact with their pet or passengers, etc. Being distracted while driving and speeding or while under the influence of alcohol greatly increase the risks of being distracted while driving. If you do not have a little bit of fear while driving, you should not drive. If you are not aware of how dangerous driving can be, then you will not focus one hundred percent of your attention on driving.

Give driving your complete and total attention. Common distractions are talking on the phone, texting, putting on makeup, arguing or fighting with passengers, reading a map or magazine, eating, looking at the landscape, daydreaming, playing with a pet or attending to a screaming or crying child. It is important to ignore your cellphone while driving. To avoid cellphone-related distractions it is helpful to turn your cellphone off before you get inside your vehicle.

Do not drive when you are under stress or experiencing extreme emotions. You should drive only when you feel emotionally stable. When experiencing extreme emotions, such as depression, anxiety, hysteria, anger, etc. your brain is focusing on and processing the matters that have caused your emotional state. This will cause you to be less aware of the surrounding traffic and road conditions. Tears caused by depression or crying can cause your vision to be cloudy or otherwise reduce your ability to see clearly. Anxiety and panic attacks can cause people to speed. Laughter and anger can lead to reckless driving and loss of control of the vehicle.

Do not ever drive when you are tired. Being sleepy, even slightly drowsy, severely diminishes attentiveness, especially when driving long distances at consistent speeds at night on the highway. Plan ahead and prepare for your drive. You know yourself and your capacities the best; if you anticipate that you are getting tired, take a short nap before starting to drive. You should pull over to a safe area and take a nap if you begin to feel tired while you are driving. Make sure to get a good night's sleep the night beforehand you plan to drive for a long distance. Some people start to feel sleepy after driving for more than one hour (these people usually have motion sickness as well). If any of this applies to you, then you should try to pull over and take a nap every thirty minutes or share driving duties with another driver. Avoid taking medications that cause drowsiness, such as sleeping pills, antihistamines, some painkillers, etc. Avoid driving long distances after having a physically or emotionally exhausting day.

Ways to Stay Alert While Driving

1. Ingesting caffeine in the form of coffee or tea, or eating sugary cookies or candy, or drinking sugary sodas and fruit juice can artificially elevate your ability to pay attention for a short period of time and may help you be better able to pay attention and stay awake while driving.

2. Keeping the temperature inside your car cool instead of warm or hot can reduce your likelihood of feeling sleepy.

3. Avoid eating a big meal before driving.

4. Listen to music that is enjoyable and upbeat and try to have a non-emotional conversation with the passenger to help you stay awake and prevent boredom.

5. Do not drive when you are mentally or physically tired because being tired will lower your ability to pay attention and focus on your driving. Driving is exhausting, especially for older people, and you should not drive more than eight hours a day (unless you are a professional driver, such as a cab driver, truck driver, etc.).

6. Do not drive if you have a health condition that can compromise your driving ability. The status of your health can affect your ability to be a good driver. Elderly people, those older than age seventy-five, become tired easily, so they should avoid driving long distances and driving alone. People who have emphysema, heart failure, COPD, etc. become fatigued or tired more easily because their brains can lack oxygen; people with these conditions should avoid long distance drives and probably shouldn't drive alone. Pain can be distracting, so if you suffer from pain or cramps, do not drive. If you are epileptic and your condition is not under control, you should avoid driving; even a small

attack that causes you to lose consciousness for only a few seconds can cause a major car accident.

7. Do not drive if you are taking certain medications or do not know how you will react to a new medication. Some medications can seriously affect your driving abilities. Narcotics, antianxiety medications and sleeping pills can cause drowsiness. In fact, professional drivers (truck drivers, pilots, etc.) are not allowed to be under the influence of these medications while working. High blood pressure medications can lower your blood pressure too much causing you to become physically tired or to have cold sweats, if this happens to you, you should not drive. Some diabetic medications can cause your blood glucose level to be too low which can temporarily weaken your cognitive skills or cause a seizure. You must be extra cautious after taking medication. Be aware that, although it is not illegal to drive under the influence of these prescription medications, they can still cause unsafe driving and lead to accidents.

8. Consistent drug and alcohol abuse can slowly damage your brain and can cause attention disorders. It is best, for all aspects of your health and safety, to limit or avoid the use of alcohol and drugs.

Other Major Causes of Traffic Injuries and Fatalities

Impaired driving caused by alcohol or drug use –alcohol-impaired drivers were involved in almost one-third of all traffic-related deaths, resulting in nearly 11,000 deaths in 2009.[7] Alcohol and drugs are poison to the brain and therefore affect our cognitive skills. If you drive under the influence you put your wallet, health and life at risk, and turn your car into a lethal weapon to yourself and those around you. Unfortunately, many people driver under the influence of alcohol or drugs and the majority of them are not caught.

Do not drink an alcoholic beverage if you have to drive soon. Although there is a legal alcohol blood content level everybody is different; some people get affected by a very little amount of alcohol and others can drink a lot without feeling anything, additionally it depends on what you are drinking, how full or hungry you are and your health conditions. If it is your first time trying a certain type of alcohol you may be surprised at how much it affects you. It is better to not take a chance.

Drugs seriously impair cognitive skills. When you are high, have not slept for a few days because of a high, or are withdrawing from drugs your brain is not functioning at its' optimal level and your ability to pay attention is poor. In recent years, far more people abuse legal drugs (such as narcotic, anti-anxiety or anti-seizure medicine) as opposed to illegal ones, especially older people whose cognitive skills and alertness can be offset by these medications.

Aggressive Driving –driving a vehicle in a way that ignores the rights or safety of other is dangerous. Intentionally taking action that disturbs other drivers, frequently changing lanes, frequently speeding up or down, or disregarding traffic laws and signals are forms of aggressive driving. If you are an aggressive driver, consider the possible long-term effects of your actions. If you are confronted or disturbed by an aggressive driver, stay calm. Do not let someone else's failure to control their emotions cause you to lose your focus on driving safely. Keep a safe distance from an aggressive driver and do not pass them unless it is absolutely necessary for you to do so. Do not respond to the other driver's threats or gestures or allow them to cause you to slow down, and if necessary, call 911.

Failure to yield and failure to use turn signals –over twenty percent of multiple-vehicle accidents result from failure to yield. Failure to yield is the second leading cause of multiple-vehicle accidents. Be patient and do not rush. Follow traffic rules, pay attention to traffic signs and use caution when checking for oncoming traffic. Failing to yield or use your turn signals is considered aggressive driving.

Tailgating –following too close behind the vehicle in front of you is the cause of almost twenty percent of all multiple-vehicle crashes. Leave enough room between you and the car ahead of you so that you will be able to stop quickly and safely. Tailgating is considered to be a form of aggressive driving.

Driving with certain health conditions –can trigger vehicle crashes. Severe body pain, dizziness, vertigo, poor vision, poorly functioning limbs, seizures and poor memory can all affect driving quality. For mature adults, it can be depressing to have to give up driving because of a health condition, but it is far safer to give up driving then it is to taking chances with your or someone else's life.

Weather Conditions –inclement weather, including rain, fog, snow, wind storms, water, snow or ice on the roads, hail, etc. can make driving more difficult or even dangerous. You need more time to be able to stop in these conditions and being able to see the road ahead of you may be very difficult or even impossible. If you cannot see clearly, you should stop driving by pulling over or getting off the road at a safe location. If you can see, but not clearly, make sure to leave extra room between you and the vehicle in front of you and make sure that you slow down enough that you will be able to stop quickly.

Motorcycles –are a very dangerous mode of transportation. Because motorcyclists have very little protection, the rates for serious and fatal injuries caused by traffic accidents are much higher than for people who ride in light passenger vehicles. Here are some common things you should know about making motorcycle riding less dangerous.

Ways to Improve Motorcycle Safety

1. Motorcyclists need tremendous balance, and it does not take much to throw them off-balance. A rock, sand, ice, and snowy or muddy roads can cause you to lose your balance.

2. Motorcycle riding can give you an adrenaline rush, a feeling that is very addictive. In order to achieve the high feeling you have to put yourself in more and more dangerous circumstances; the more you crave it, the more danger you put yourself in.

3. Riding motorcycles have various effects on your health. The noise from the loud engine and the wind can weaken and damage your hearing; wearing ear plugs can help combat hearing loss. If you ride a motorcycle around cars and trucks, then you will inhale toxins. In cold temperatures, the wind can cause stiff and painful joints, which can increase your chance of developing body inflammation.

4. Although not all states require an adult to wear a helmet while riding a motorcycle, it is much smarter to wear a helmet (the same goes for when you ride a dirt bike or bicycle). I had a patient who was in a dirt bike crash and because he was not wearing a helmet he experienced permanent brain damage and paralysis.

5. Wear leather clothes while riding a motorcycle. Leather clothing blocks harsh winds and can protect you from road burn if you crash.

6. Wear a good pair of windproof glasses. The proper glasses can protect your eyes from wind irritation, bugs, sand and rocks.

Some people are perfectly healthy and are very good drivers, yet they still get into accidents. In reality, you are only in control of how *you* drive, not how others drive. Because of this, you have to be a good, defensive driver in order to ensure the safety of yourself and others.

Ways to Be a Defensive Driver

1. While driving, remain aware of the vehicles around you. Watch the car in front of you and keep enough distance from it, note to yourself whether or not the vehicle stays in the center of its lane, if it is off center, you should keep even more distance from it.

2. Make sure the vehicle behind you is not too close to your car, if it is, change lanes or pull over in order to let the car pass.

3. Make sure to not hover in the blind spot of a car that is next to you.

4. Even if you have the right of way at a sign or a stoplight, double check to make sure there are no vehicles coming or people walking in the crosswalk.

5. Do not stop abruptly at stop signs and signal lights or try to run through yellow lights.

6. Do not stop over the recommended stopping line so that you do not block pedestrians or other cars that are trying to turn and must pass by your car to do so.

7. Avoid driving in bad weather conditions as much as possible. No matter how good of a driver you are, poor weather conditions can make the road a dangerous place for you. The chance of experiencing a crash increases when weather conditions are bad. It is important to keep extra distance between yourself and other drivers in poor weather conditions.

8. Use extra caution around the holidays, especially New Year's Eve. Holidays tend to increase the amount of people driving under the influence of alcohol.

9. If you have poor vision, do not drive at dusk or at night.

10. If you know you have existing medical conditions or are taking medications

that can decrease your driving ability, don't take chances; do not drive.

Lack of fear and responsibility –if you have absolutely no fear of driving, then you should not drive. When you drive, you are responsible not only for your life, but also the lives of your passengers and the lives of other people on the road. Try to remember that every time you drive, you are taking on a huge responsibility. Here are a few points to keep in mind about preventing accidents.

1. People tend to be more fearful of driving after they experience a vehicle crash, and usually drive more cautiously after having been in a crash. Sometimes, these people gradually lose their sense of responsibility and end up having more vehicle crashes. If you remain aware of the responsibility you have as a driver, then you will decrease your chances of causing a crash.

2. Learn about what has caused other people's crashes. Take time to talk about what caused other driver's accidents or study accident statistics and causes online so that you can gain wisdom from other people's mistakes.

3. Read or study your state's traffic crash reports at least once a year and check updated traffic reports every time you head out to drive in traffic. This can help you be more cautious and aware of potentially dangerous driving areas or conditions where you live.

4. Take good care of your car. Make sure to check the tires often and keep everything well-maintained, don't ignore or put off any important car repairs.

It is highly likely that at some point in your life, you that you will be involved in a vehicle collision either as a driver or as a passenger. It's not uncommon for people to experience more than one crash in their lifetime. Nearly all people in developed and most developing countries ride in vehicles from birth, so throughout a person's lifetime, only a small percentage of people will not be involved in a vehicle crash of some type. The current statistics in the United States estimate that your yearly chance of being involved in an accident is 1 in 32.[8] Let us remember, most vehicle crashes are preventable accidents, that is, they are caused by people's mistakes and can be prevented or avoided. For your and other people's safety, health and quality of life –please drive cautiously and responsibly.

Chapter Eleven

Unnecessary Prescriptions

What You Need to Know to Prevent Yourself from Being Overmedicated

For the average American, taking prescription and over-the-counter drugs (including supplements) has become an integral part of their day to day lives. In general, about one half of all Americans are taking at least one prescription drug in any given month.[1] These medications are made from processed, highly concentrated chemicals, the majority of which have serious side effects that can cause severe health problems. Unfortunately, most of the people who take medication do not need to take medication. I have found the following common reasons to describe why people allow themselves to be overprescribed medication, that is, why people take unnecessary medication.

Inability to access necessary information –the majority of people do not always know how or where to access the information they need to make informed health decisions. Most people are unaware that most of the medications that doctors prescribe are not necessary. There are alternative approaches that may have slower results, but can help prevent you from having the problem for the rest of your life. Doctors tend to present medication as the best and, in some cases, the only treatment. Patients are not generally encouraged to seek information about alternative treatments when they seek care for their health concerns, so they simply don't know about all of the treatment options available to them.

Unrealistic faith in medication –people are often made to feel that taking a pill will provide immediate and effective relief. Antibiotics, vaccines and other drugs have become widely used and effective since the middle of the twentieth century. Because of this, people have developed a mindset that has caused them to believe that medication can solve all ailments. Most people who take medication do so more out of mental reliance than actual physical need. This is why placebo trials (sugar pills) often show surprising rates of improvement, especially with psychiatric medications.[2, 3]

Using medicine as a security blanket –people often feel reassured about their health condition when they take medication. Many people think that health ailments cannot be addressed or fixed without medication. They also feel that as long as they take their medication, then they have adequately protected their health and may even feel that they have done everything they possibly can to secure their health. This is why older patients take multiple medications (in some cases, from my experience, up to twenty different medications each day).

The quick fix –some people want their health conditions to be resolved quickly and without too much effort. Prescribing medication is convenient for both doctors and patients. Doctors are able to be more economical with their time and see more patients if they can simply write a prescription. Most doctors do not take time to figure out what exactly is causing their patients' physical or mental problems, so they often prescribe medication without identifying the cause of health problems. If you or your doctor cannot identify the cause of your problem, then there is a high chance that taking medication as a treatment is unnecessary or not the proper treatment. For patients, swallowing a pill for physical and mental problems seems like a fast and easy fix in comparison to developing willpower and self-discipline to bring about lifestyle changes. Taking pills as opposed to enacting lifestyle changes is easier and requires less effort than natural approaches to health.

Withdrawal –some people are afraid to experience unpleasant side effects that may be associated with stopping their medication. Many people continue taking medication because when they try to stop, they experience negative and unpleasant withdrawal symptoms and the condition that they are taking the medication for worsens. For example, when someone stops taking hormone replacement therapy (such as birth control pills or thyroid hormone replacements), the previous syndrome becomes worse than before. Hormone medications compete with the body's natural production of these same hormones, so when you stop taking these medications it takes time for your body to be able to produce its own hormone supply and sometimes is never able to start making its own supply again.

Addiction to medication –often people develop physical or physiological addictions to medication. Many medications are extremely addictive, especially antidepressants, sleeping and narcotic pills; a lot of people end up addicted to these medications. For example, narcotic pain medication is made from opiates that share the same origins as heroin and are just as addictive as the illegal form of the drug.[4] Trying to stop narcotic medication can be very difficult, and, in some cases, even dangerous. Additionally, after taking narcotic medication many people pursue the narcotic high, either through illegally obtaining prescription medication or through the use of heroin. Prescription painkiller overdosing is the leading cause of accidental death in the United States, having surpassed traffic accidents.[5] Furthermore, these medications affect sleep, and can easily lead to depression, which can cause the person to start taking antidepressants. This can start the cycle of taking more medication to address the side effects of the initial medication. Each time new medication is added, there is a potential to develop a new set of side effects and health problems. There are far safer ways to treat and manage pain than through highly addictive narcotic medications.

Fear of change or failure to commit to change –some people are hesitant to educate themselves and make needed changes to preserve their health. There is so much information online and at the library about diseases and health ailments that it is likely you will find out more about your problems by doing your own research than from listening to your doctor (who has very limited time and is probably not willing to thoroughly explain the cause or source of your health problems). For example, a patient of mine had severe psoriasis. His doctor gave him the immunosuppressor prednisone and various other medications, but his condition did not improve. Finally, his wife began to do research about his condition and she found that food allergies, usually citrus fruit and dairy, can trigger psoriasis. He stayed away from these foods and his psoriasis completely disappeared. Later, he tried to eat cheese and orange juice, but saw immediately that his psoriasis flared up. Clearly, these substances were the cause of his problem. Through education, he was able to learn how to avoid the causes of his disease and successfully control his psoriasis without the use of medication.

Insurance covers medication –some people believe that taking prescription medications is an affordable way for them to treat their conditions. Although monetarily it may seem more cost-effective to take medication, in the end these medications can cause more health problems, which leads to more doctor visits, medications and procedures, all of which insurance companies usually require deductibles and copayments, not to mention required monthly premium payments that increase the more you use your medical insurance. As a person's health condition deteriorates or becomes more complicated from the growing number of side effects, more and more medical procedures are required, costing more money (and possibly lost income from missed work) and more time. That is why medical bills are the number one cause of bankruptcy in America.[6] How much more cost effective it is for us to learn how to preserve and maintain our health so we don't need to take medications.

Sometimes, it is necessary to temporarily take medications. For example, when a person has a serious infection, injury, experiences shock, heart attack, stroke, etc. administered medication can be life-saving and the only option available. However, long-term medication usage is, most of the time, unnecessary. If you find yourself having to take medication, then you should be aware of all the side effects and understand your health condition as thoroughly as possible so that you can accurately judge whether or not the medication is working for you. Also, you need to educate yourself about what other treatment options are available or how lifestyle changes can successfully eliminate your health concerns.

It is important to not place all of your faith in medications. You should continually educate yourself about your condition so that you can understand what the best treatment is for your condition. It is a good idea to visit chiropractors, naturopaths, acupuncturists, massage therapists, etc. (all of which usually provide a free initial consolation) to get their opinion about your health ailment. By gathering as much information from as many viewpoints and opinions as possible, you can make the best, educated decisions on how to manage, treat and prevent your health problems and severely cut down your chance of taking unnecessary medication.

It may be very difficult to accept the fact that many doctors unnecessarily prescribe medications. But, once you understand the reasons why they may do so, it starts to make sense why Western medicine relies so heavily on pharmaceuticals. From my experience, I have found some common reasons why medication is prescribed on a regular basis.

Prescribing medication saves time and increases clinic productivity. The more patients that doctors are able to see, the more revenue they are able to earn. So, the quicker they move on to the next patient, the more productive their day will be. Doctors are frequently overbooked, and, more often than not, make you wait for a long time before seeing them. The fastest way to treat patients is through prescribing medication. In one hospital I visited there was a sign on the wall that stated each patient was allowed to ask the doctor only two questions and could not take up more than seventeen minutes of the doctor's time. Clearly, in this kind of environment, medication is the easiest and quickest way to treat patients.

Lack of communication with your doctor can increase your chance of being overprescribed medication. As mentioned above, doctors are often overbooked and very busy. If they have a policy that prevents a patient from even asking more than two questions in the course of an office visit, then how is it possible to build an effective and caring doctor/patient relationship – one that will be based on making decisions that are best for your health and not time or profits? If your doctor does not take the time to get to know you and your medical history, then you have a high chance of being prescribed unnecessary medication. For example, a doctor may give you medication for a symptom or health concern that is, in fact, just the side effect of another medication you are taking. A patient of mine had a sleep disorder that was caused by taking antidepressant medications. When she visited her doctor for her sleep problems, her doctor automatically gave her a prescription for sleeping medication. However, she knew for a fact that her sleeping disorder was caused by the antidepressant medication because before taking the antidepressant she did not have any sleeping problems. If you have good communication with your doctor, then the likelihood that you will be prescribed unnecessary medication will be greatly reduced.

Doctors are trained to treat diseases and illnesses with pharmaceutical medications. Just as acupuncturists will treat you with acupuncture, because that is what they are trained to do; a doctor will treat you with medication because doctors are trained to prescribe medication. The majority of Western medicine physicians earnestly believe that medication is the best way to treat most health issues. Unfortunately, few doctors will investigate what is causing their patients' problems and instead simply treat the symptoms with medication.

Doctors try to please patients. Many people go to their doctor expecting to be given a prescription, so doctors will often prescribe medication just to satisfy their patients and maintain a good rapport with them.

Pharmaceutical companies invest in building relationships with physicians. Many pharmaceutical companies give doctors free samples to hand out to patients; and incentives to learn about and prescribe their medications. Recently, these activities have become more regulated, but pharmaceutical companies still have a huge influence on the type and amount of medications doctors prescribe to their patients.

Here Are a Couple of Examples of Commonly Prescribed Unnecessary Medications

Two-thirds of all prescription refills at pharmacies are for sleeping pills, antidepressants, narcotics and antianxiety medicines.[7, 8] Most of these disorders can be managed and treated properly through alternative, less harmful, approaches. For example, many factors can cause sleep disorders. You know yourself the best, so you have the best chance of accurately identifying what causes your sleep disorder. Once you identify the cause, you can adjust your lifestyle in order to achieve the quality and quantity of sleep you need. Sleep medications can have disruptive and unpleasant side effects such as daytime drowsiness, snoring or sleep apnea. Also, many of these medications are extremely addictive. As your body adjusts to the medication, you may end up having to take more and more to achieve the initial results you experienced as well. When you stop these medications, you may experience severe withdrawal syndrome, which can make it even more difficult to for you to be able to fall asleep.

A patient of mine had a lower than normal thyroid hormone count, so his doctor gave him a prescription for hyperthyroid medication, regardless of the fact that he did not have any symptoms. The patient began taking the medication, and soon after he could not sleep. His heart began to race and he was having heart palpitations. He immediately stopped taking the medication. A few months later, he had his thyroid re-checked and the reading was normal. Even years later, he is still fine without taking thyroid medication. If he had continued to take the hormone supplements his body would have developed a dependency on it, and he would be less able to naturally produce thyroid hormones. Clearly, he did not need to take this medication, but the doctor prescribed it to him anyway. Millions of people are prescribed unnecessary medication, and take it to the point where it actually becomes destructive as opposed to being helpful.

The best way to treat Type II Diabetes is to, first and foremost, change lifestyle and dietary habits. As you exercise and eat better, your condition will improve and possibly reverse. Unfortunately, many people think that the main treatment for diabetes is medication. Some people believe that if they are diabetic (adult-onset Type II Diabetes), then they absolutely must take medication. Some people even use medication as an excuse to keep their self-destructive lifestyle habits. It is important to remember that over 28,000 unintentional poisonings occur each year from improper prescription and over-the-counter drug use.[9] Medical reactions result in over one and a half million emergency room visits in the U.S. each year. Emergency room visits caused by reactions to medicine are second only to trips to the E.R. caused by automobile accidents.[10, 11] Accidental drug deaths do not include acute deaths caused by chronic prescription drug use such as liver failure, kidney failure or heart attack related to the long-term use of narcotics, pain relievers, anti-inflammatories, etc. For example, when the Food and Drug Administration removes a drug from the market because it has been shown to cause an increased risk of death or illnesses that lead to death, those deaths are not included in the number of yearly unintentional drug deaths.

Before beginning a new medication, you should study about what is causing your illness. Take advantage of learning about what other alternatives are available. If you have an illness caused by life and dietary choices, such as high blood pressure, you may choose to take medication for the short-term, but commit yourself to long-term lifestyle change with the goal of self-managing without needing medication, or better yet, manage your life now so that you never have to worry about having to take medications for lifestyle caused diseases.

Unnecessary Surgeries

What You Need to Know Before Going Under the Knife

Unnecessary surgeries are ones that, afterwards, do not make you feel better, make you feel worse, or do not improve or resolve your health problem. Most surgeries can be very damaging and invasive to your body, so it is best to pursue alternative methods before having a drastic surgery. If surgery is not performed as a last resort, then it is highly likely that undergoing surgery is not necessary. When necessary, surgery can be responsible for saving people's lives, but when performed unnecessarily, it can actually create more health problems or make existing problems worse.

No matter how good the surgeon is and how smoothly the surgery goes, a surgery involves cutting tissue, which causes deliberate injury to the body. Surgery can have many complications. Surgery can lead to infections. When your body is cut open, your chance of contracting an infection is high. If things go wrong in major surgeries, like brain and heart surgeries, there can be serious consequences. Your body's natural response to being cut is to create a blood clot in order to stop the bleeding. Blood clots, a common post-surgical trauma, can cause stroke, heart attack or collapsed lung.

Anesthesia used in surgeries can be very dangerous, and, in some cases, can cause death.[12, 13] The use of anesthesia may also lead to chronic body aches and pain, as well as permanent brain damage, including the early onset of dementia.[14] Surgery can cause long-term pain near incision areas due to nerve damage and scar-tissue buildup.

Any area of your body that is operated on will never feel the same as it did before undergoing surgery. If you have an emergency, life-threatening condition that only surgery can resolve, then it is most likely necessary. But, if you have a chronic condition, then you have time to research your condition and figure out the root causes. When you take the time to do this, you will be able to determine the true causes of your illness and you will be able to make the best decisions in order to restore and preserve your health. In most cases you may find that much less drastic measures can be taken to successfully treat your problem.

There Are Many Reasons Why Surgery Rates in America Are So High

Failure to learn all you can about your medical condition and care. If you do not educate yourself and go to your doctor without an understanding of your situation, then you are essentially giving your doctor the power and responsibility to make decisions for you. However, what is in your doctor's best interest may not always be what is in your best interest. For example, I had a patient who was scheduled to have hip replacement surgery. His surgeon told him that his hip joint was "bone-on-bone" and that his cartilage had worn off. He had just had his other hip replaced the previous year. He felt that his first replacement hadn't been successful. He had been suffering from stiffness and pain ever since his hip had been replaced. This led him to decide to change his mind and cancel his surgery. He decided he would wait as long as he could before he would have surgery again. A few months later, his hip pain (in the hip that he was told needed to be replaced) went completely away for no reason that he could think of. Now, he feels no pain or stiffness in that hip joint, but he feels constant pain in his replaced hip. He spends time regretting his first hip surgery now and often says that he wonders if the surgery had really been necessary and how he would have felt if he hadn't of had undergone it. He regrets it every day.

Another patient I have was in her late 70's when her doctor recommended that she have surgery to treat her lower back pain and sciatica. He told her that if she did not undergo surgery that her pain would become disabling and she would be in a wheelchair in less than two years. Now, fourteen years later, she laughs when she tells me how her doctor lied to her. Now, in her nineties, she is still walking. She just gave up driving last year, but is living on her own and happy that she was able to protect herself enough to understand that doctors are not always right. Doctors cannot predict the outcome or always be right about what is going to happen if you do or don't undergo surgery.

One of my patients had knee pain and his doctor had recommended that he get his knee replaced. The doctor told him that there were no other options for him to address his knee pain. The man had never undergone surgery and was terrified of the idea of having an operation. He decided that he would get a second opinion. That was when I met him. In fact, the majority of my patients come to me as a "last resort" before undergoing surgery. After he received two acupuncture sessions, he felt better and decided that he would not undergo surgery. Four visits later, he was walking without pain even though the doctor had told him that his knee joint was "bone-on-bone" and now he wonders why his doctor wanted him to have his knee replaced.

Another patient of mine was in her mid-thirties. She had mid and lower back pain. Her doctor told her that she had a uterus disorder that was causing her back pain. She underwent a hysterectomy. Her back pain didn't improve, so her doctor told her that she had cysts on her ovaries that were causing her back pain. So, she had her ovaries removed. Her back pain did not go away. She came to see me. I discovered that her back pain was coming from improper posture while sitting at work. I trained her how to sit properly and improve her posture and I used acupuncture therapy to treat the inflammation in her back. After six sessions, her back pain was gone. This makes her wonder how accurate her doctor's diagnoses were before it was recommended that she have surgery.

The purpose of my sharing these stories with you is to provide you with examples of why it is important to always look for treatment alternatives. Surgery should be reserved as the last choice to be used only after nothing else has worked. I encourage you to keep an open mind to try new and alternative medical therapies. As I mentioned earlier, most health care practitioners will provide you with a second opinion at no cost. Again, take advantage of opportunities to learn as much as you can about all aspects of available health care choices.

Fear that something life-threatening is wrong with you. A patient of mine had been having headaches and was advised to have an MRI. His doctor found a tumor in his brain and informed him that most likely it was cancerous. The man decided to immediately undergo brain surgery to have the tumor removed. As it turned out, the tumor was not cancerous. Unfortunately, one side of his body was paralyzed by the surgery and he is now permanently disabled. His fear of having cancer was so extreme that it caused him to make a rash decision that he will have to suffer from for the rest of his life. Even though the threat of brain cancer is very severe and frightening, it is important to calm down and gather as much information as possible before making any decisions.

Surgery is often viewed as a quick fix for health ailments. A patient I consulted with had bursitis (commonly known as "frozen shoulder"). I told her that physical therapy or acupuncture therapy would be able to heal her bursitis, but that it would take about six months of regular therapy. However, she wanted a quicker fix, so she decided to have surgery. The operation helped her regain a few degrees of her range of motion (flexibility), but she still was required to receive physical therapy about three times per week for almost six months after the surgery. Not only that, but her shoulder never felt quite the same again. She told me that she felt a constant, dull pain in her shoulder that just never went away. Unfortunately, it is almost impossible for surgery-related pain to ever fully go away. It is most likely that she will suffer from pain in her shoulder for the rest of her life.

Surgery is covered by insurance. I had a twenty-two year old patient who had been suffering with extremely painful periods for a few years. Her doctor recommended that she have a hysterectomy. She had a good job that provided health insurance coverage that would pay for her procedure in full. She had delayed making a decision as to whether or not she would have the surgery, but when she became concerned that she would lose her job, she decided to have the hysterectomy just in case she wouldn't have insurance benefits to cover it later. After the surgery, she ended up with incontinence and hormone disorders (menopausal syndrome) that she now has to suffer from on a daily basis. She will have to manage these conditions every day for the rest of her life, not to mention the fact that she will never be able to have her own children.

I have seen so many people over the years choose surgery as their first treatment choice because they have insurance benefits that pay for surgery. While insurance carriers continue to routinely deny coverage for alternative therapies that are not only cheaper in the short-term, but save countless amounts of expenses in the long-run from additional treatments required for side effects such as more surgeries, frequent doctor visits and life-long dependency on prescription medications. Surgery is not only expensive for insurance companies, but for the patient as well. Often, the costs are much greater than just financial losses. Free time and quality of life is more often than not diminished after undergoing surgery from time wasted by being in discomfort or pain, returning to the doctor and not feeling well enough to participate in normal activities.

The majority of people believe that surgery is a cure-all. People who have had one successful surgery are more likely to undergo surgery again. A patient of mine had twenty-seven surgeries after having one successful knee-replacement surgery. After so many surgeries, he was suffering from pain in multiple places in his body. It made him wonder how much of his pain has been caused by his surgeries. On the other hand, I had a patient who had moderately severe lower back pain for a few months. He had just retired and loved to play golf. His doctor recommended that he have back surgery. He made an appointment and was getting off of the hospital's elevator when a man, who was much younger than him and hunched over in pain, was leaving the surgeon's office. After talking to the man, he discovered that the man had just undergone back surgery and was experiencing much more pain than before he had the surgery, and was now facing having to undergo more surgeries. My patient told me that after he talked to this man, he got back in the elevator, left the hospital and never returned. He has never had to have surgery; he plays golf almost daily, travels with his wife and enjoys a very high quality of life. He receives acupuncture two or three times a year and only if he feels some pain acting up in his back or if he slightly injures or overuses his muscles. He has saved tens of thousands of dollars and added potentially years of quality of life to his "golden years" because he was able to make a decision based on long-term results instead of seemingly cheaper, quicker fixes.

Applying for and keeping disability benefits. I had a patient who, after having thirteen back surgeries, went from having mild back pain now and then to having a much worse and chronic pain condition. After all of those surgeries, he became disabled. I have had patients tell me how their doctors' only solution for their disability is surgery, especially for back injuries. I often find that they continue to undergo surgeries because they feel pressure to follow their doctors' orders. Unfortunately, some people undergo surgery under their doctors' recommendation so that they may qualify for disability or maintain their disability status. Do not automatically trust that undergoing surgery is necessary because you have been injured in an auto or work-related accident. If you don't have a good reason to undergo surgery – other than that it is covered by your insurance –you may not start out disabled, but you may very well end up disabled.

Surgeries are promoted in our healthcare system. First of all, surgery and all the expensive equipment it requires, is an extremely profitable business. Surgeries create profits for doctors, hospitals, pharmaceutical and medical equipment companies and hospitals. The reality is that the better insurance coverage you have, the higher your chance of undergoing unnecessary surgery will be. Many doctors believe that surgery is the best and fastest way to solve your health problems.

Another reason surgery is promoted is because doctors who are experienced in surgery or accustomed to referring patients to surgeons will always suggest surgery before recommending any other approaches. General practitioners and other health care providers are very concerned with the potential liability associated with not sending a patient to a surgeon or specialist. It is very sad that the medical system in our country has been forced into a position that prevents physicians from using all of the available tools to help a patient preserve and regain health. Instead, doctors must first be concerned with protecting themselves from malpractice lawsuits and accusations of improper care.[15] Clearly, if they simply send you home with a prescription or send you to the surgeon, they are able to greatly reduce their personal risk because they have done what is expected of them. The best way to avoid unnecessary surgery is to discuss your situation with your doctor from the vantage point that you are an informed patient who is aware of and understands all of your options and that you are not willing to make rash decisions or expect your doctor to be solely responsible for your health.

Chapter Twelve

What Now and What Next? Turning Common Sense into Practical Life Changes

The Journey to Your Best Health Starts with You

The path to achieving good health is paved with learning the correct health knowledge, self-discipline and action. The first step requires you to educate yourself so that you will be able to make well-informed decisions. Accumulating medical knowledge to become a doctor is not easy, but learning general health knowledge and ideas does not require any medical training whatsoever. Remember that investing in your health is one of the best things you will ever do for yourself (and those love you).

Taking charge of your health is the single most important and rewarding decision you will ever make because:

1. Medical expenses are the leading cause of personal financial crises and bankruptcy in America.[1]

2. Without good health, life can become worthless. Regardless if you are wealthy or poor, successful or unsuccessful, bad health affects everyone. Nothing puts a stop to living your ideal life faster than poor health.

3. Bad health does not only affect you. It also affects those around you, especially your family. Illness places immeasurable burdens not only on yourself, but on those you love.

Overall, maintaining good health is the foundation you need in order to be able to enjoy everything you have or want in life. So, the more you invest in good health and learn about how to take proper care of yourself, the better quality life you will be able to live. You can use this book as a foundation to learn how to properly invest in and build personal health and well-being. If this book has taught you only one thing that has helped you to change your lifestyle or the way you approach your personal health care, then I have achieved my goal. However, I know that that this book is not perfect and that one man's wisdom is not all that you need. I simply hope that this book has helped to put yourself on a good path and launched you in the right direction.

Because of the internet, there is a lot of unreliable and misleading health information readily available, but there is useful health information available online as well, so it is important to use your discernment and investigate any claims made by a company or organization. Make sure that you check with multiple sources before you decide to agree with or disagree with health claims made. Consider the sources you use before accepting research findings. Consider the factors in your own life that may interplay with diet, exercise and environmental choices you make. Just like there is healthy food and junk food. There is also healthy information and junk information.

Learn as Much as You Can from Various Sources and Trust Your Judgment Before Accepting Health Information

There are a lot of diet programs, groups and supplements that claim they can help you lose weight. The truth is that cutting down caloric intake and increasing exercise is the healthiest, cheapest and most effective way to lose weight. However, cutting down to consuming too few calories is not healthy either. You need to find a sustainable balance and make sure you get enough nutrition. One common example of people searching for a quick-fix without fully understanding their individual needs is the popularity of "detox" dieting.

Many of my patients have asked me for herbs to help them detox their body without figuring out how to stop putting toxins into their bodies in the first place. Some examples of perpetual toxin exposure include consuming too many calories, eating preserved, fried, grilled or smoked foods, and eating foods that have been produced to ensure a long shelf-life. Beverages such as alcohol, prepared juices, sodas (regular or diet) and even teas (black, green, herbal, etc.) that have been sprayed with pesticides and herbicides add toxins to your body.

Medications are chemicals that can be extremely toxic. Many of the side effects of prescription medications are caused by the toxins they release into your body. Supplements (vitamins, minerals, beverages, powdered proteins, etc.) can overload your body. There can be toxic substances in your environment such as cigarette smoke and pollution. Anything put on your skin such as makeup, lotion, perfume and cologne can be absorbed into your body. This is why it is extremely important to use discernment when choosing the types of products you allow to be used in your home and on your body.

The body also naturally produces toxins such as sweat, feces and urine. The longer waste stays in your colon, the more toxins stay (reabsorbed) in your body. The longer uric acid (from urine) stays in your body, the more toxic it is for your body because it can cause inflammation in your arteries leading to atherosclerosis. If you are dehydrated, your body will not be able to flush uric acid out. Cells produce toxins. Cells –like individual human beings – eat, breathe and produce waste which needs to be transported via the bloodstream, through exercise, in order to be excreted from the body.

If you understand the different ways that toxins are created in the body, you can take the necessary steps to help detox your body and cut down the amount of toxins your body has to get rid of. For example, you can stop eating toxic foods, stop drinking toxic drinks, use your nose and cognitive skills to create a healthy environment, put less chemical products on your skin, make sure you have regular bowel movements, drink plenty of water and do plenty of exercise in order to promote blood circulation and rid the body of toxic cell waste.

If you put fewer toxins into your body you will not need to detox your body later on. Many advertised products claim to be able to effectively detox the body, either through supplements, juices, colonics, various miracle substances, diets and programs. But, if you have common sense about toxins, learn how to detox yourself and keep yourself detoxed; you can save your time and money. More so, most of these miracle detox substances can actually put more toxins in your body, so it is important that you educate yourself in order to make the proper choices.

Hopefully this book has helped you develop a new perspective on how to cultivate, achieve and sustain good health. It is my goal for you that this new perspective will help you make healthier choices and move forward on your path to optimal health.

Another important step towards optimal health is self-discipline. It is possible that you already knew some of the information presented in this book, but because you were unaware of your lack of self-discipline, you may not have acted on your knowledge. Most of the information I have presented may be new to you, but it is important that you develop the self-discipline necessary to take what you have learned seriously and act on it. Without self-discipline, health knowledge and information is absolutely useless. Disciplining yourself is, of course, easy to say and hard to do. Every day people fight battles with themselves to try to do what is best for their health instead of what they want. Remember making good decisions not only helps you achieve good health, but can influence the people closest to you by directly encouraging them through your actions to make positive changes in their lives as well.

You can bring a horse to water, but you cannot force the horse to drink. I have brought you to the waters of good health, but in order to achieve good health, you have to take action and drink –that is, do the hard work! Many people try to take shortcuts by swallowing pills, taking supplements, undergoing surgery, etc. These approaches will not change your lifestyle and, therefore, your health problems will not truly be treated. Your condition will not be healed until you make the changes required to prevent re-injuring or causing more harm to your body.

I invite you to give me feedback about this book; whether through questions, concerns or sharing your own sensible ideas with me and the Common Sense Health community. We can work together to create a healthier America. The most important step you can take is to figure out what is causing your illness. After you have discovered the root cause or causes of your illness, you will be able to take the necessary steps (including educating yourself about your illness, learning how to make lifestyle changes in order to reduce your illness and prevent it from getting worse, reduce your chances of re-injuring yourself and what treatment options you may need to seek) to allow your body to recover and heal itself. With all of the information available on the internet and at libraries, you can educate yourself with knowledge as the first step of placing your health in your own hands.

Now that you have learned simple steps to change your lifestyle as a way to heal and prevent ailments, you can learn how to treat existing health concerns without medications or potentially unsafe medical interventions. Please look for my book entitled *True Answers –Finding and Treating the Causes of Common Illnesses* which provides a detailed guide on how to use preventive health for specific illnesses –from head to toe, inside and outside of your body. I explore and explain the causes of various illnesses and pain conditions and help you understand how to help yourself heal your health problems. My goal is to assist you in learning all you can about taking care of yourself through knowledge.

You can find resources for the Common Sense Health community at www.bambridgemedicalarts.com. There you will find the tools you need to assist your learning process, educational materials and health care references based on a variety of topic and up to date information on the latest global health news and reports from traditional and alternative treatment perspectives.

Bambridge Medical Arts, Inc. is a health education company that was created to educate you on how to prevent illness before you get sick and how to find and treat the cause of your illnesses. I sincerely believe that you do not have to be a medical doctor in order to learn how to properly take care of and preserve your individual health.

We offer an educational series based on traditional Chinese medicine that may be performed at home or work on yourself or your family using simple techniques based on Chinese acupressure and other therapy methods. This series of self-care health videos teaches you how to find the cause of specific health ailments and how to use traditional Chinese therapies to treat them as well as methods to prevent them from recurring. You can learn from these videos how to incorporate preventative lifestyle changes so that you never have to worry about developing certain ailments at all. As is often said and I have found to be true, "An ounce of prevention is worth a pound of cure."

Visit Bambridge Medical Arts at www.bambridgemedicalarts.com to access our educational portal. This site provides links to all consumer health information and services we provide including the latest news about preventative health, our self-care treatment series at www.10minutes2health.com, my private practice clinic information at www.wangmedicalinc.com, and www.bambridgeonlinecourses.com (which is dedicated to training and assisting professional health care providers expand their practice treatment tools by using theories and methods based on traditional Chinese medicine).

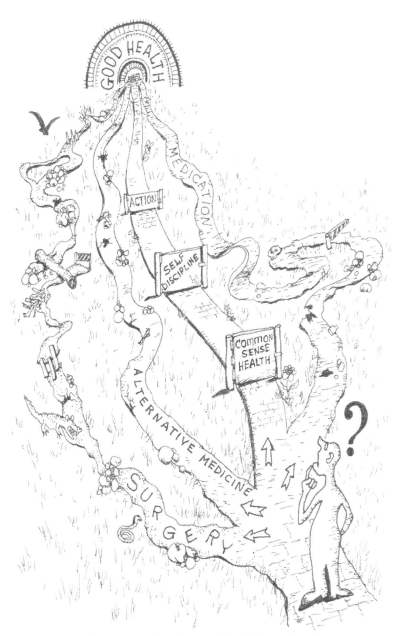

There are no shortcuts to achieving good health. Learn how to overcome
health hurdles through personal education and action.

10minutes2health.com is dedicated to consumer health care education. The core of the program is based on a series of videos and downloadable eBooks that provide in-depth information on preventative care and acupressure techniques that can be used to address specific ailments at home or work without the use of medicine or expensive equipment.

Some of the current titles include:

Macular Degeneration & Eye Care which teaches you how to apply simple acupressure techniques to reduce symptoms caused by allergies such as watery and itchy eyes, how to reduce eyestrain caused by computer or other types of work that require nearsighted-focus and how to reduce and reverse vision loss caused by macular degeneration. Most of us know someone who is suffering from age-related eye loss. There are ways to address this condition without surgery or medications.

Frozen Shoulder & Shoulder Pain teaches you how to use exercise and massage to relieve shoulder pain and frozen shoulder (also known as fifty year old shoulder). Most of us experience some type of shoulder pain or injury as we age. Learn how to use your own hands to heal your condition and avoid unnecessary shoulder surgery.

Migraine & Headache Relief provides a simple to follow acupressure application that can be used anytime, anywhere to immediately reduce the pain caused by most types of headaches and migraines, including headaches caused by other health disorders.

TMJ Syndrome is designed to relieve jaw and head pain caused by excessive chewing, grinding teeth, jaw joint injury and more. The program is designed to relieve the syndrome and teaches you how to prevent it from recurring without using equipment.

Carpal Tunnel Syndrome is an incredible program that has been effective in helping a variety of people reduce and reverse their work-related repetitive stress injuries. If you drive, keyboard, write, sew, work in retail, garden, ride a bicycle, bake, cook, paint, practice artwork, perform work (dentists, checkers, massage therapists, computer programmers, etc.) or engage in an activity that requires the use of your hands, you may have already experienced the disruptive effects caused by wrist pain and the associated shoulder, arm, hand and finger pain and numbness. This program teaches you how to address and relieve this syndrome and how to change your activities so that you can prevent re-injury and continue to enjoy your work and hobbies.

Whiplash & Neck Pain is a comprehensive program that teaches you how to relieve neck pain caused by whiplash syndrome, poor posture, injuries, fibromyalgia and more. It will also teach you how to change your sleeping, sitting and working positions to prevent neck pain and injuries. If you have neck pain or whiplash syndrome, this program will guide you on how to prevent your symptoms from getting worse and prevent re-injury.

Sinus Allergies & Pain is designed to teach you how to use acupressure techniques to relieve sinus allergies, post-nasal drip, watery nose, sneezing, pain and inflammation caused by sinus infection and more. You will learn how to reduce your risk of getting sinus allergies by removing potential allergens from your life as well.

Digestive Disorders teaches you effective ways to relieve the symptoms caused by food allergies, digestive diseases & pain and menstrual pain. Recently, Crohn's disease, celiac disease, food allergies, disrupted & imbalanced digestion, irregularity, upset stomach and ulcers have become more and more common. Most of us know someone who suffers from heartburn, indigestion, food allergies or some other type of intestinal discomfort. Digestive disorders can disrupt your ability to enjoy your daily life. Learn how to not only treat existing conditions, but also how to prevent flare-ups. The program includes an in-depth discussion of how to change your diet to meet your individual digestive needs and concerns.

Traditional Chinese Cupping Therapy is an interesting ancient therapy that isn't yet well known in the West. This program evaluates the different types of cups used in cupping therapy including bamboo, glass and plastic cups and how to effectively apply them to the body for effective relief of asthma, sciatica, arthritis, joint pain and muscle injury. Cupping therapy is commonly used in acupuncture clinics when needle therapy isn't appropriate for the patient.

Chinese Moxa & Heat Therapy teaches you how to use a variety of heat-producing natural products (including moxa herbs) to address a variety of common ailments including warts, skin viruses, shingles, stress-related hair loss, joint pain and more.

10minutes2health.com's blog covers a variety of health topics, including the latest news in medical care and changes around the globe. You can find everything you need to stay connected to all of the information you need to stay in control of your health care. Consumer resources including how to get a second opinion and how to be your own health advocate are provided as well.

Thank you for letting me to share this information with you. It is my primary goal is to provide the tools you need to empower yourself to take care of yourself through health education and support. Please, let us know how we can help you.

"Taking Responsibility for Your Own Health is the Best Way to Achieve Good Health."

                                                      -Feng-Ling Wang

References Cited by Chapter

Chapter One

World Health Organization, "Data Repository," [http://apps.who.int/ghodata/] (2011) List of global statistics on major factors that affect life expectancy and quality of life.

Chapter Two

Kendall, Cyril W.C.; Emam, Azadeh; Augustin, Livia S.A.; Jenkins, David J.A., "Resistant Starches and Health," (May-June 2004) *AOAC Journal*, Volume 87, Issue 3 pages 769-774 (This issue of The Association of Official Analytical Chemists' Journal contains several detailed articles discussing the roles of resistant starches in the diet.)
[2] Natural Resources Defense Council, "Facts about Pollution from Livestock Farms," (January 13, 2011) [http://www.nrdc.org/water/pollution/ffarms.asp]
[3] National Cancer Institute at the National Institutes of Health, "Acrylamide in Food and Cancer Risk," (July 29, 2008) [http://www.cancer.gov/cancertopics/factsheet/Risk/acrylamide-in-food]
[4] A very helpful nutritional content tool can be found at [http://nutritiondata.self.com/tools/compare/welcome?returnto=/tools/compare]. This site provides detailed nutritional facts on several types of whole and processed foods and allows you to compare the nutritional content of foods.
[5] National Soybean Research Laboratory [http://www.nsrl.illinois.edu/soy_benefits.html]
[6] Cordle, C., "Protein Allergy: Incidence and Relative Severity," *The Journal of Nutrition* May 1, 2004 Volume 134 Issue 5 pages 1213-1219
[7] World Health Organization, "Diabetes (Fact Sheets)," (August 2011) [http://www.who.int/mediacentre/factsheets/fs312/en/]
[8] Science Daily, "Charred Meat May Increase Risk Of Pancreatic Cancer," (April 21, 2009) [http://www.sciencedaily.com/releases/2009/04/090421154327.htm]
[9] National Center for Biotechnology Information, affiliated with the National Institutes of Health, provides a variety of public medicine articles that may be accessed at ncbi.nlm.nih.gov, , that discuss detailed research the health risks causes by cooking gases. Go to [http://www.ncbi.nlm.nih.gov/pubmed] and enter "cooking with gases" in the "pubmed" search bar to find articles. Pubmed refers to

public medicine, that is, medical issues that affect the community, a group of people or the public at large.

10 Food and Agriculture Organization of the United Nations "Non-meat Ingredients" is a detailed list provided by the that outlines additives that are approved and commonly added to the meat-based food supply.
[http://www.fao.org/docrep/010/ai407e/AI407E06.htm] Information about other important food supply ingredients can be found at fao.org.
11 Wang, Y. & Shan, J., "Safety of Food Chain Ensured at Source," (February 23, 2010) China Daily News
[http://www.chinadaily.com.cn/usa/2010-02/23/content_11016161.htm] Although the FDA has banned the use of Clenbuterol in animals, meat that is imported may contained these additives. A list of food additives banned by the FDA can be found at farad.org (Food Animal Residue Avoidance Databank)
12 Mitchell, G.A. & Dunnavan, G., "Illegal use of beta-adrenergic agonists in the United States," (January 1998) Journal of Animal Science [http://jas.fass.org/content/76/1/208]
13 Union of Concerned Scientists, "Prescription for Trouble: Using Antibiotics to Fatten Livestock," (2012)
[http://www.ucsusa.org/food_and_agriculture/science_and_impacts/impacts_industrial_agriculture/prescription-for-trouble.html]
14 Rogers, I.S., Northstone, K., Dunger, D., Cooper, A., Ness, A. & Emmett, P.M., "Diet throughout Childhood and Age at Menarche in a Contemporary Cohort of British Girls," (June 2010) Research Paper for Public Health Nutrition, Volume 13, Issue 12 pages 2052-2063
http://journals.cambridge.org/action/displayAbstract?fromPage=online&aid=7924542&fulltextType=RA&fileId=S1368980010001461]
15 Environmental Protection Agency, "Nitrites and Nitrates," TEACH Chemical Summary accessed at
[epa.gov/teach/chem_smm/Nitrates_summary.pdf. epa.gov/teach] provides in-depth findings about the presences and use of nitrites and nitrates in a variety of food applications.
16 Food Safety and Inspection Service (of the United States Department of Agriculture), "USDA Issues Final Rule on Meat and Poultry Irradiation," (December 1999)
[http://www.fsis.usda.gov/Oa/background/irrad_final.htm]
17 Food and Drug Administration, "Bad Bug Book 2nd Edition Foodborne Pathogenic Microorganisms and Natural Toxins Handbook," (April 3, 2012) can be downloaded at fda.gov. This handbook provides a guide for common organisms found in the food supply that may cause illness.

[http://www.fda.gov/food/foodsafety/foodborneillness/foodborneill
nessfoodbornepathogensnaturaltoxins/badbugbook/default.htm]
[18] Go to [http://ars.usda.gov/main/site_main.htm?modecode=12-35-
45-00] and click on "Search the USDA National Nutrient Database for
Standard Reference" or download a search tool to your computer. The
information provides the composition of vegetables. (May 16, 2012)
The information is based on comprehensive research conducted by the
Unites States Department of Agriculture (USDA).
[19] Robertson, D.S., "The Function of Oxalic Acid in the Human
Metabolism," (September 1, 2011) *Clinical Chemistry & Laboratory
Medicine*, Volume 49, Issue 9 pages 1405-1412
[20] Baba, A., Catoi, C., "Comparative Oncology," (2007) Bucharest: The
Publishing House of the Romanian Academy, Chapter
2,Carcinogenesis [http://www.ncbi.nlm.nih.gov/books/NBK9552/]
[21] American College of Allergy, Asthma & Immunology, "Shellfish
Allergy," (2010) [http://www.acaai.org/allergist/allergies/Types/food-
allergies/types/Pages/shellfish-allergy.aspx]
[22] American Academy of Allergy, Asthma & Immunology, "Allergy
Statistics," (2012) [http://www.aaaai.org/about-the-
aaaai/newsroom/allergy-statistics.aspx]
[23] Raloff, J., "No Peanuts for Your Peanut," (a blog entry for the web
edition of Science News, Magazine of the Society of Science and the
Public) (December 2009)
[http://www.sciencenews.org/view/generic/id/9197/title/Food_for_
Thought__No_Peanuts_for_Your_Peanut]
[24] The Food Allergy and Anaphylaxis Network, "Tree Nuts," (March
28, 2012) [http://www.foodallergy.org/page/tree-nut-allergy]
[25] Food Standards Agency, "Peanuts During Pregnancy, Breastfeeding
and Early Childhood," (August 24, 2009)
[http://www.food.gov.uk/safereating/allergyintol/peanutspregnancy]
[26] University of Michigan Health System, "Choking Prevention,"
(March 2011)
[http://www.med.umich.edu/yourchild/topics/choking.htm]
[27] Raloff, J., "No Peanuts for Your Peanut," (a blog entry for the web
edition of Science News, Magazine of the Society of Science and the
Public) (December 2009)
[http://www.sciencenews.org/view/generic/id/9197/title/Food_for_
Thought__No_Peanuts_for_Your_Peanut]
[28] Medline Plus, U.S. Library of Medicine (NIH), "Lactose
Intolerance," (April 16, 2012)
[http://www.nlm.nih.gov/medlineplus/ency/article/000276.htm]

29 BBC News, "Timeline: China Milk Scandal," (January 25, 2010) [http://news.bbc.co.uk/2/hi/7720404.stm]

30 Kirk, J., "Commonly Used Antibiotics on Dairies," [http://www.vetmed.ucdavis.edu/vetext/INF-DA/Antibiotics-Dairies.pdf]

31 American College of Allergy, Asthma and Immunology, "Egg Allergy," (2010) [http://www.acaai.org/allergist/allergies/Types/food-allergies/types/Pages/egg-allergy.aspx]

32 Picciano, M.F., Office of Dietary Supplements, (NIH)"Who Is Using Dietary Supplements and What are They Using?," (November 27, 2005) [http://ods.od.nih.gov/pubs/fnce2005/M%20F%20Picciano-Who%20Is%20Using%20Dietary%20Supplements%20and%20What%20are%20They%20Using.pdf]

33 Breastcancer.org, "Women Often Take Antioxidants During Breast Cancer Treatment," (June 8, 2009) [http://www.breastcancer.org/tips/new_research/20090608b.jsp]

34 Centers for Disease Control and Prevention, "Hemochromatosis Facts," July 5, 2011) [http://www.cdc.gov/ncbddd/hemochromatosis/facts.html]

35 University of Cincinnati Health News, "Hot Liquids Release Potentially Harmful Chemicals in Polycarbonate Plastic Bottles," (January 30, 2008) [http://healthnews.uc.edu/news/?/6387]

36 Natural Resources Defense Council, "Bottled Water," (April 25, 2008) [http://www.nrdc.org/water/drinking/qbw.asp]

37 BBC News, "Why Is Drinking Too Much Water is Dangerous," (January 15, 2007) [http://news.bbc.co.uk/2/hi/6263029.stm]

38 Ballantyne, C., "Strange but True: Drinking Too Much Water Can Kill," (June 21, 2007) Scientific American [http://www.scientificamerican.com/article.cfm?id=strange-but-true-drinking-too-much-water-can-kill]

39 Johns Hopkins Medicine, "Caffeine Withdrawal Recognized as a Disorder," (September 29, 2004) [http://www.hopkinsmedicine.org/press_releases/2004/09_29_04.html]

40 Sheps, S., Mayo Clinic, "High Blood Pressure Q & A: "How Does Caffeine Affect Blood Pressure?," (October 21, 2011) [http://www.mayoclinic.com/health/blood-pressure/AN00792]

41 U.S. Department of Health and Human Services, National Kidney and Urologic Diseases Information Clearinghouse (NKUDIC), "What I Need to Know About Kidney Stones," (September 2, 2010) [http://kidney.niddk.nih.gov/kudiseases/pubs/stones_ez/]

[42] National Resources Defense Council (NRDC), "Chemicals in Plastic Bottles: How to Know What's Safe for Your Family," (May 2008) [http://www.nrdc.org/health/bpa.pdf]

[43] NRDC, "Environmental Issues: Health, Coffee, Conservation, and Commerce in the Western Hemisphere," [http://www.nrdc.org/health/farming/ccc/chap4.asp]

[44] Bente, H., Carlsen, M., Phillips, K., Bohn, S., Holte, K., Jacobs, D. Jr., Blomhoff, R., "Content of Redox-active Compounds (ie, antioxidants) in Foods Consumed in the United States 1,2,3," (2006) American Society for Clinical Nutrition [http://ajcn.nutrition.org/content/84/1/95.full#cited-by] (View tables of foods with highest antioxidants per serving.)

[45] National Resources Defense Council (NRDC), "Chemicals in Plastic Bottles: How to Know What's Safe for Your Family," (May 2008) [http://www.nrdc.org/health/bpa.pdf]

[46] Greenpeace, "Banned Pesticides Found in Teas Produced by Popular Chinese Tea Brands," (April 11, 2012) [http://www.greenpeace.org/eastasia/press/releases/food-agriculture/2012/chinese-tea-banned-pesticides/]

[47] Environmental Working Group (EWG), "Bisphenol A: Toxic Plastics Chemical in Canned Food: Consumer Tips to Avoid BPA Exposure," [http://www.ewg.org/bisphenol-a-info] (This site contains several articles that discuss the use of BPA in consumer products.)

[48] University of Cincinnati Health News, "Hot Liquids Release Potentially Harmful Chemicals in Polycarbonate Plastic Bottles," (January 30, 2008) [http://healthnews.uc.edu/news/?/6387]

[49] Healthy Child, Healthy World –Chemical Encyclopedia, "polycyclic aromatic hydrocarbons (PAHs)," [http://healthychild.org/issues/chemical-pop/polycyclic_aromatic_hydrocarbons/] (The information listed can apply to adults as well.)

[50] CDC, "Food Safety at CDC –Some Foods and Germs," (May 10, 2012) [http://www.cdc.gov/foodsafety/specific-foods.html]

[51] Food Standards Australia New Zealand, "Acrylamide and Food," (September 2011) [http://www.foodstandards.gov.au/consumerinformation/acrylamideandfood.cfm]

[52] Eat Safe, "Oil Abuse," (June 22, 2012) [http://eatsafe.co.za/site/index.php?option=com_content&view=article&id=49:oil-abuse&catid=40:articles&Itemid=74]

[53] National Cancer Institute at the National Institutes of Health, "Chemicals in Meat Cooked at High Temperatures and Cancer Risk,"

(October 15, 2010)
[http://www.cancer.gov/cancertopics/factsheet/Risk/cooked-meats]
54 Raloff, J., "Carcinogens in the Diet," (a blog entry for the web edition of Science News, Magazine of the Society of Science and the Public)[
http://www.sciencenews.org/view/generic/id/5890/title/Carcinogens_in_the_Diet]
55 National Cancer Institute at the National Institutes of Health, "Chemicals in Meat Cooked at High Temperatures and Cancer Risk," (October 15, 2010)
[http://www.cancer.gov/cancertopics/factsheet/Risk/cooked-meats]
56 The Cancer Project, "Cancer Facts –Meat Consumption and Cancer Risk [http://www.cancerproject.org/survival/cancer_facts/meat.php]
57 National Cancer Institute at NIH, "Diet and Diseases," (February 26, 2004)[http://www.cancer.gov/newscenter/entertainment/tipsheet/diet-related-diseases]

Chapter Three

1 Mayo Clinic, "Performance-enhancing Drugs: Know the Risks," (December 23, 2010)
[http://www.mayoclinic.com/health/performance-enhancing-drugs/HQ01105]
2 Center for Young Women's Health, Children's Hospital Boston, "Sports and Menstrual Periods: The Female Athlete Triad," (May 21, 2010) [http://www.youngwomenshealth.org/triad.html]
3 Ganbari, Z., Manshavi, F., Mina, J., "The Effect of Three Months Regular Aerobic Exercise on Premenstrual Syndrome," (December 2008) *Journal of Family & Reproductive Health,* Volume 2, Issue 4 pages 167-171
4 American Pregnancy Association, "Effects of Exercise on Pregnancy," (June 2011)
[http://www.americanpregnancy.org/pregnancyhealth/effectsofexerciseonpreg.html]
5 Johns Hopkins Medicine, "Get Moving to Protect Your Prostate," (January 27, 2009)
[http://www.johnshopkinshealthalerts.com/alerts/enlarged_prostate/JohnsHopkinsEnlargedProstateHealthAlert_2904-1.html]
6 Cancer Research UK, "Risks and Causes Of Penile Cancer," (June 1, 2012) [http://cancerhelp.cancerresearchuk.org/type/penile-cancer/about/risks-and-causes-of-penile-cancer]

[7] Nayal, Schwarzer, Klotz, Heidenreich and Engelmann, "Transcutaneous Penile Oxygen Pressure During Bicycling," (1999) *British Journal of Urology International,* Volume 83 pages 623–625

[8] Verret, C., Guay, M., Berthiaume, C., Gardiner, P., Béliveau, L., "A Physical Activity Program Improves Behavior and Cognitive Functions in Children with ADHD: An Exploratory Study," (January 2012) *Journal of Attention Disorders,* Volume 16, Issue 1 pages 71-80

[9] Chaddocka, L., Ericksonb, K., Prakashc, R., "A Neuroimaging Investigation of the Association Between Aerobic Fitness, Hippocampal Volume, and Memory" (2010) *BrainResearch,* 1358 pages 172-183 [http://kch.illinois.edu/research/labs/neurocognitive-kinesiology/files/Articles/Chaddock_2010_ANeuroimagingInvestigationOf.pdf]

[10] Please study information about sports safety and protecting your children from injuries. You can find numerous research-based articles and information at [www.safekids.org] (search: "sports safety guide" and "safety basics" [www.aans.org] (search: sports injuries in children) and [www.osha.gov] (search: "children at play"). Learn the risks based on your children's individual needs and then take the necessary precautions suggested to protect them.

[11] Centers for Disease Control and Prevention (CDC) "Falls Among Older Adults: An Overview" (February 29, 2012) cdc.gov [http://www.cdc.gov/HomeandRecreationalSafety/Falls/adultfalls.html]

[12] National Ski Areas Association, "Facts About Skiing/Snowboarding Safety," (September 1, 20122) [http://www.nsaa.org/nsaa/press/NSAA-Facts-Ski-SnowB-Safety-9-11.pdf]

[13] CDC, "Snowmobile Fatalities --- Maine, New Hampshire, and Vermont, 2002—2003," (December 19, 2003) *MMWR,* Volume 52, Issue 50 [http://www.cdc.gov/mmwr/PDF/wk/mm5250.pdf]

[14] Environment and Human Health, Inc., "The Harmful Effects of Vehicle Exhaust" [http://www.ehhi.org/reports/exhaust/summary.shtml]

[15] Agency for Toxic Substances & Disease Registry, CDC, "Toxic Substances Portal – Chlorine," (March 3, 2011 [http://www.atsdr.cdc.gov/toxfaqs/tf.asp?id=200&tid=36]

[16] James, R., "A Brief History of the Marathon," (October 30, 2009) *Time,* [http://www.time.com/time/nation/article/0,8599,1933342,00.html]

[17] Verret, C., Guay, M., Berthiaume, C., Gardiner, P., Béliveau, L., "A Physical Activity Program Improves Behavior and Cognitive Functions

in Children with ADHD: An Exploratory Study," (January 2012) *Journal of Attention Disorders*, Volume 16, Issue 1 pages 71-80

[18] Alzheimer's Association, "Brain Injury May More Than Double Dementia Risk in Older Veterans," (July 18, 2011) Press Release from Alzheimer's Association International Conference July 16-21, 2011 Paris, France [http://www.alz.org/aaic/monday_1230amct_news_release_brain_injury.asp]

[19] National Ski Areas Association, "Facts About Skiing/Snowboarding Safety," (September 1, 20122) [http://www.nsaa.org/nsaa/press/NSAA-Facts-Ski-SnowB-Safety-9-11.pdf]

[20] CDC, "Snowmobile Fatalities --- Maine, New Hampshire, and Vermont, 2002—2003," (December 19, 2003) *MMWR*, Volume 52, Issue 50 [http://www.cdc.gov/mmwr/PDF/wk/mm5250.pdf]

[21] American Alpine Club, "Accidents in North American Mountaineering Statistical Tables," [http://www.americanalpineclub.org/p/anam-statistics] Provides a list of mountaineering accidents by year (for most years) from 1951 to present.

Chapter Four

"Link Between Fast Food and Depression Confirmed" (March 30, 2012) sciencedaily.com

[2] Chawla, J., Suleman, A., Carcione, J., "Neurologic Effects of Caffeine," (November 21, 2011) [http://emedicine.medscape.com/article/1182710-overview]

[3] Tyas, S., National Institute on Alcohol Abuse and Alcoholism, "Alcohol Use and the Risk of Developing Alzheimer's Disease," [http://pubs.niaaa.nih.gov/publications/arh25-4/299-306.htm]

[4] Mayo Clinic, "Schizophrenia: Symptoms" (January 27, 2012) [http://www.mayoclinic.com/health/schizophrenia/DS00196/DSECTION=symptoms]

[5] Nemours, "ADHD: Tips to Try," [http://kidshealth.org/teen/school_jobs/school/adhd.html#a_Tips_to_Try]

[6] Dranov, P. "Tired? Depressed? Check Your Thyroid" *American Health* (May 1994)

[7] Sandel, M.E., Weiss, B., Ivker, B., "Multiple Personality Disorder: Diagnosis After a Traumatic Brain Injury," (June 7, 1990) *Physical Medicine and Rehabilitation*

[8] Family Advocacy, Wright-Patterson Air Force Base, Family Advocacy, "How to Recognize Family Maltreatment," (August 7, 2007) [http://www.wpafb.af.mil/library/factsheets/factsheet.asp?id=9391]

[9] See information provided about alcohol abuse in Chapter Nine.

[10] National Center for Health Statistics, CDC, Pratt, L., Brody, D., Gu, Q., "Antidepressant Use in Persons Aged 12 and Over: United States, 2005–2008," (October 11, 20011) NCHS Data Brief Number 76 [http://www.cdc.gov/nchs/data/databriefs/db76.pdf]

[11] National Institute on Drug Abuse, "Drug Facts: Prescription & Over-the-Counter Medications," (May, 2012) [http://www.drugabuse.gov/publications/drugfacts/prescription-over-counter-medications]

[12] Centers for Disease Control and Prevention, "Health, United States, 2011," (2011) [http://www.cdc.gov/nchs/data/hus/hus11.pdf#100][13] You can do a search for the side effects of specific medications at [http://www.drugs.com/sfx/]. This site is designed for consumer use.

[14] Mayo Clinic Staff, "Seasonal Affective Disorder (SAD) Definition," (September 22, 2011) [http://www.mayoclinic.com/health/seasonal-affective-disorder/DS00195]

[15] Nielsen, "State of the Media: March 2011 U.S. TV Trends by Ethnicity," (2011) [http://www.nielsen.com/content/dam/corporate/us/en/reports-downloads/2011-Reports/State-of-the-Media-Ethnic-TV-Trends.pdf]

[16] Sewards, T., Sewards, M., "Fear and Power-Dominance Drive Motivation: Neural Representations and Pathways Mediating Sensory and Mnemonic Inputs, and Outputs to Premotor Structures," (2002) *Neuroscience and Biobehavioral Review*, Volume 26, Issue 5, pages 553-579

[17] Bruehl, S., Burns, J., Chung, O., Chont, M., "Pain-related Effects of Trait Anger Expression: Neural Substrates and the Role of Endogenous Opioid Mechanisms," (2009) *Neuroscience and Biobehavioral Reviews*, Volume 33, Issue 3 pages 475-491

[18] Pridmore, S., Turnier-Shea, Y., "Medication Options in the Treatment of Treatment-resistant Depression," (2004) *Australian & New Zealand Journal of Psychiatry*, Volume 38, Issue 4, pages 219-225

[19] Lam, R., "Adjunctive Medication Strategies for Treatment-resistant Depression," (2011) *Canadian Journal of Psychiatry*, Volume 56, Issue 6 pages 315-316

[20] Centers for Disease Control and Prevention, "Therapeutic Drug Use," (May 18, 2012) [http://www.cdc.gov/nchs/fastats/drugs.htm]

[21] Helpguide.org, Kemp, G., Smith, M., DeKoven, B., Segal, J., "Play, Creativity, and Lifelong Learning

Why Play Matters for Both Kids and Adults," (February 2012)
[http://www.helpguide.org/life/creative_play_fun_games.htm]

Chapter Five

Centers for Disease Control and Prevention, "Are You Getting
Enough Sleep?," (August 31, 2009)
[http://www.cdc.gov/Partners/Archive/Sleep/]
2 Blask, D., "Melatonin, Sleep Disturbance and Cancer Risk," (2009)
Sleep Medicine Reviews Volume 13 pages 257–264
[http://depts.washington.edu/epidem/Epi583/2009_11_06/Blask_Me
latonin&Cancer.pdf]
3 American Pregnancy Association, "Sleep Positions During
Pregnancy" (March 2007)
[http://www.americanpregnancy.org/pregnancyhealth/sleepingpositio
ns.html]
4 American Pregnancy Association, "Sleep Positions During
Pregnancy" (March 2007)
[http://www.americanpregnancy.org/pregnancyhealth/sleepingpositio
ns.html]

Chapter Six

Judson R, Richard A, Dix DJ, Houck K, Martin M, Kavlock R, et al.,
"The Toxicity Data Landscape for Environmental Chemicals. Environ
Health Perspect," (2009) [http://dx.doi.org/10.1289/ehp.0800168]
2 World Health Organization, "The Top Ten Causes of Death," (June
2011) [http://www.who.int/mediacentre/factsheets/fs310/en/]
3 World Health Organization, "Cancer," (February 2012)
[http://www.who.int/mediacentre/factsheets/fs297/en/]
4 World Health Organization, "Indoor Air Pollution and Health,"
(September 2011)
[http://www.who.int/mediacentre/factsheets/fs292/en/]
5 California Department of Public Health, "Chemicals Known or
Suspected to Cause Cancer of Reproductive Toxicity," (December 1,
2010)
[http://www.cdph.ca.gov/programs/cosmetics/Documents/chemlist.
pdf]
A starting point for consumer research can be found at
Safecosmetics.org. This group provides links to published articles from
a variety of sources about the use and regulation of carcinogenic
ingredients in consumer body care products.

[6] United States Food and Drug Administration (FDA), "Report to Congress on the FDA Foreign Offices," (February 2012) [http://www.fda.gov/Food/FoodSafety/FSMA/ucm291803.htm]

[7] National Cancer Institute at the National Institutes of Health, "Hair Dyes and Cancer Risk," (August 10, 2011) [http://www.cancer.gov/cancertopics/factsheet/Risk/hair-dyes]

[8] World Health Organization, "Mercury Present in Skin Lightening Products," (2011) [http://www.who.int/ipcs/assessment/public_health/mercury_flyer.pdf]

[9] FDA, "Lipstick and Lead: Questions & Answers," (April 12, 2012) [http://www.fda.gov/Cosmetics/ProductandIngredientSafety/ProductInformation/ucm137224.htm?utm_campaign=Google2&utm_source=fdaSearch&utm_medium=website&utm_term=coal%20in%20lipstick&utm_content=1#q7]

[10] FDA, "Color Additives and Cosmetics," (April 26, 2007) [http://www.fda.gov/ForIndustry/ColorAdditives/ColorAdditivesinSpecificProducts/InCosmetics/ucm110032.htm]

[11] How Stuff Works, "The Chemistry of Cosmetics —Coal Tar Colors — Suspected Cancer Culprit," [http://science.howstuffworks.com/the-chemistry-of-cosmetics-info2.htm] This site provides an easy to understand explanation of the use of color additives in cosmetics.

[12] National Cancer Institute, "Benzene-Exposed Workers in China," [http://dceg.cancer.gov/reb/research/other/4]

[13] National Cancer Institute at the National Institutes of Health, "Formaldehyde and Cancer Risk," (June 10, 2011) [http://www.cancer.gov/cancertopics/factsheet/Risk/formaldehyde]

[14] Medline Plus, A Service of the U.S. National Library of Medicine, National Institutes of Health, "Cloth Dye Poisoning," (February 28, 2012) [http://www.nlm.nih.gov/medlineplus/ency/article/002784.htm]

[15] Heller, K., Pringle, C., "Economic Impact Analysis (EIA) for the Fabric Coatings NESHAP," (March 2001) [http://www.epa.gov/ttnecas1/regdata/IPs/Fabric%20Coatings_IP.pdf]

[16] Environmental Protection Agency (EPA), "An Introduction to Indoor Air Quality (IAQ) Volatile Organic Compounds (VOCs)," (May 3, 2012) [http://www.epa.gov/iaq/voc.html]

[17] EPA, "OPPT Chemical Fact Sheets Nitrobenzene Fact Sheet: Support Document (CAS No. 98-95-3)," (February 1995) [http://www.epa.gov/chemfact/nitro-sd.pdf]

[18] Medline Plus, A Service of the U.S. National Library of Medicine, National Institutes of Health, "X -Plain Dust Mite Allergy Reference Summary," (December 18, 2010) ["http://www.nlm.nih.gov/medlineplus/tutorials/allergiestodustmites /id039204.pdf] You can participate in an interactive tutorial provided by the U.S. National Library of Medicine, National Institutes of Health at [http://www.nlm.nih.gov/medlineplus/tutorials/allergiestodustmites/ htm/index.htm]

[19] Environment and Human Health, Inc.,"The Harmful Effects of Vehicle Exhaust," [http://www.ehhi.org/reports/exhaust/summary.shtml]

[20] National Cancer Society, "Diesel Exhaust," (June 12, 2012) [http://www.cancer.org/Cancer/CancerCauses/OtherCarcinogens/Po llution/diesel-exhaust]

[21] World Health Organization, "Diesel Engine Exhaust Carcinogenic," (June 12, 2012) Go to: [http://www.who.int/en/] and search "diesel]

[22] Chilcott, R., Health Protection Agency, "Compendium of Chemical Hazards: Diesel," (2006) [http://www.who.int/ipcs/emergencies/diesel.pdf]

[23] Alavanja, M., Bonner, M.; "Occupational Pesticide Exposures and Cancer Risk: A Review," (2012) *Journal of Toxicology and Environmental Health*, Part B: Critical Reviews, Volume 15, Issue 4, pages 238-263

[24] World Health Organization, "Air Quality and Health," (September 2011) [http://www.who.int/mediacentre/factsheets/fs313/en/]

[25] Canadian Centre for Occupational Health & Safety, "What are the Effects of Dust on the Lungs?," (April 18, 2002) [http://www.ccohs.ca/oshanswers/chemicals/lungs_dust.html]

[26] Please see Chapter Two for more information about this topic.

Chapter Seven

National Heart, Lung and Blood Institute, NIH, "What is Raynaud's?," (February 1, 2011) [http://www.nhlbi.nih.gov/health/health-topics/topics/raynaud/]

[2] Mayo Clinic Staff, "Seasonal Affective Disorder (SAD) Definition," (September 22, 2011) [http://www.mayoclinic.com/health/seasonal-affective-disorder/DS00195]

[3] World Health Organization, "International Travel and Health 2010," Chapter 3 Environmental Health Risks [http://www.who.int/ith/ITH2010chapter3.pdf]

[4] World Health Organization, "International Travel and Health 2009," Chapter 5 Infectious Diseases of Potential Risk for Travelers [http://www.who.int/ith/ITH2009Chapter5.pdf]
[5] Mayo Clinic Staff, "Heatstroke," (September 2, 2011) [http://www.mayoclinic.com/health/heat-stroke/ds01025/dsection=symptoms]

Chapter Eight

Centers for Disease Control Prevention, "Cigarette Smoking Among Adults and Trends in Smoking Cessation --- United States," (November 13, 2009) *MMWR*, Volume 54, Issue 44 pages 1227-1232 [http://www.cdc.gov/mmwr/preview/mmwrhtml/mm5844a2.htm]
[2] Centers for Disease Control and Prevention, "Adult Cigarette Smoking in the United States: Current Estimates," (March 14, 2012) [http://www.cdc.gov/tobacco/data_statistics/fact_sheets/adult_data/cig_smoking/]
[3] Centers for Disease Control and Prevention, "Health Effects of Cigarette Smoking," (January 10, 2012) [http://www.cdc.gov/tobacco/data_statistics/fact_sheets/health_effects/effects_cig_smoking/]
[4] National Cancer Institute at the National Institutes of Health, "Harms of Smoking and Health Benefits of Quitting," (January 12, 2011) [http://www.cancer.gov/cancertopics/factsheet/Tobacco/cessation]
[5] Siemiatycki J., Krewski D., Franco E., Kaiserman M., "Associations Between Cigarette Smoking and Each of 21 Types of Cancer: A Multi-site Case-control Study," (June 1995) *International Journal of Epidemiology*, Volume 24, Issue 3 pages 504-514 [http://www.ncbi.nlm.nih.gov/pubmed/7672889]
[6] Centers for Disease Control and Prevention, "Adult Cigarette Smoking in the United States: Current Estimates," (March 14, 2012) [http://www.cdc.gov/tobacco/data_statistics/fact_sheets/adult_data/cig_smoking/]

Chapter Nine

National Highway Traffic Safety Administration (NHTSA), "Impaired Driving," [http://www.nhtsa.gov/Impaired]
[2] NHTSA, "Secretary Peters Launches National Drunk Driving Enforcement Campaign and Encourages Judicial Branch Help," (August 20, 2007) [http://www.nhtsa.gov/About+NHTSA/Press+Releases/2007/Secret

ary+Peters+Launches+National+Drunk+Driving+Enforcement+Cam
paign+and+Encourages+Judicial+Branch+Help]

[3] You can read "2006 Traffic Safety Annual Assessment –Alcohol-
Related Fatalities," at [http://www-
nrd.nhtsa.dot.gov/Pubs/810821.PDF]

[4] National Digestive Diseases Information Clearinghouse (NDDIC) A
Service of the NIDDK at the National Institutes of Health,
"Cirrhosis," (February 21, 2012)
[http://digestive.niddk.nih.gov/ddiseases/pubs/cirrhosis/#cause]

[5]Department of Health & Human Services Substance Abuse and
Mental Health Services Administration –Fetal Alcohol Spectrum
Disorders (SAMSHA FASD Center for Excellence), "Stop and Think.
If You're Pregnant, Don't Drink," (May 30, 2012)
[http://fasdcenter.samhsa.gov/index.cfm]

[6] Lupton, C., SAMSHA FASD Center for Excellence, "The Financial
Impact of Fetal Alcohol Syndrome," (2003)
[http://fasdcenter.samhsa.gov/publications/cost.cfm]

[7] Kendall, R., PubMed, U.S. National Library, NIH, "Alcohol and
Suicide," (1983) Summary of Article appearing in *Substance Alcohol
Actions Misuse*," Volume 4, Issue 2-3 pages 121-127
[http://www.ncbi.nlm.nih.gov/pubmed/6648755]

[8] National Institute of Arthritis and Musculoskeletal & Skin Diseases,
"Q&A about Osteonecrosis (Avascular Necrosis," (August 2011)
[http://www.niams.nih.gov/health_info/osteonecrosis/#b]

[9] National Institute on Drug Abuse, "Drug Facts: Prescription & Over-
the-Counter Medications," (May, 2012)
[http://www.drugabuse.gov/publications/drugfacts/prescription-over-
counter-medications]

[10] Arizona Department of Health Services, "DBHS Practice Protocol
Older Adults: Behavioral Health Prevention, Early Intervention, and
Treatment," (August 24, 2011) [
http://www.azdhs.gov/bhs/guidance/olderadult.pdf]

[11] Centers for Disease Control and Prevention, "CDC Grand Rounds:
Prescription Drug Overdoses — a U.S. Epidemic," Morbidity and
Mortality Weekly Report (MMWR), (January 13, 2012)
[http://www.cdc.gov/mmwr/preview/mmwrhtml/mm6101a3.htm]

[12] National Drug Intelligence Center, "The Impact of Drugs on
Society," National Drug Assessment 2006 (January 2006)
[http://www.justice.gov/ndic/pubs11/18862/impact.htm]

[13] United Nations Office on Drugs and Crime (UNODC), "Economic
and Social Consequences of Drug Abuse and Illicit Trafficking," (1998)
[http://www.unodc.org/pdf/technical_series_1998-01-01_1.pdf]

14 UNODC, "The Social Impact of Drug Abuse," (World Summit for Social Development, Copenhagen, March 6-12, 1995) [http://www.unodc.org/pdf/technical_series_1995-03-01_1.pdf]

Chapter Ten

Merriam-Webster, "Merriam-Webster's Collegiate Dictionary, 11th Edition," Springfield, MA: Encyclopedia Britannica, (2008)
2 National Safety Council (NSC), FAQ: "What is the deadliest mode of transportation?" [http://www.nsc.org/news_resources/Resources/res_stats_services/Pages/FrequentlyAskedQuestions.aspx]
3 U.S. Census Bureau, "Statistical Abstract of the United States," (2012) [http://www.census.gov/compendia/statab/2012/tables/12s1103.pdf]
4 Center for Disease Control and Prevention (CDC), "Injury Prevention: Motor Vehicle Safety, (August 4, 2011), [http://www.cdc.gov/motorvehiclesafety/]
5 NSC, Speeding and Highway Safety: The U.S. Department of Transportation's Policy and Implementation Strategy," (1997) [http://www.nhtsa.gov/people/injury/enforce/shpolicy.htm]
6 Distraction.gov, "What Is Distracted Driving?," (2012) [http://www.distraction.gov/content/get-the-facts/facts-and-statistics.html] This government-sponsored website provides comprehensive data about distracted driving and how to avoid it.
7 CDC, "Injury Prevention & Control: Motor Vehicle Safety, Impaired Driving: Get the Facts," (October 18, 2011) [http://www.cdc.gov/MotorVehicleSafety/Impaired_Driving/impaired-drv_factsheet.html]
8 U.S. Department of Transportation National Highway Traffic Safety Administration, "Analysis of Fatal Motor Vehicle Traffic Crashes and Fatalities at Intersections, 1997 to 2004," (February 2007) [www-nrd.nhtsa.dot.gov/Pubs/810682.PDF]
9 U.S. Department of Transportation National Highway Traffic Safety Administration, "Analysis of Fatal Motor Vehicle Traffic Crashes and Fatalities at Intersections, 1997 to 2004," (February 2007) [www-nrd.nhtsa.dot.gov/Pubs/810682.PDF]
10 U.S. Department of Transportation, "Traffic Safety Facts 2009," [http://www-nrd.nhtsa.dot.gov/Pubs/811402.pdf]

Chapter Eleven

Centers for Disease Control and Prevention, "Therapeutic Drug

Use," (May 18, 2012) [http://www.cdc.gov/nchs/fastats/drugs.htm]

[2] American Cancer Society, "What Is the Placebo Effect?," (August 23, 2010) [http://www.cancer.org/Treatment/TreatmentsandSideEffects/Treat mentTypes/placebo-effect]

[3] Loranger A., Prout C., White M., "The Placebo Effect in Psychiatric Drug Research," *Journal of the American Medical Association*, (1961) Volume 176, Issue 11 pages 920-925

[4] National Institute on Drug Abuse, "Drug Facts: Prescription & Over-the-Counter Medications," (May, 2012) [http://www.drugabuse.gov/publications/drugfacts/prescription-over-counter-medications]

[5] Centers for Disease Control and Prevention, "Policy Impact: Prescription Painkiller Overdoses," (December 19, 2011) [http://www.cdc.gov/homeandrecreationalsafety/rxbrief/].

[6] Himmelstein, D., Thorne, D., Warren, E., Woolhandler, S., "Medical Bankruptcy in the United States, 2007: Results of a National Study" (2009) *The American Journal of Medicine*, Volume 122, Issue 8 pages 741-746

[7] Centers for Disease Control and Prevention, "Health, United States, 2011," (2011) [http://www.cdc.gov/nchs/data/hus/hus11.pdf#100]

[8] This is information I have personally collected from several pharmacists I have personally interviewed on this specific topic. Of the 5 pharmacists I questioned, all 5 told me that two-thirds of the orders they fill are for sleeping pills, antidepressants, narcotics or antianxiety medications. Two pharmacists told me that their "best-seller" is Zolpidem, a sleep aid.

[9] Centers for Disease Control and Prevention, "Policy Impact: Prescription Painkiller Overdoses," (December 19, 2011) [http://www.cdc.gov/homeandrecreationalsafety/rxbrief/]

[10] U.S. Department of Health & Human Services, AHRQ, "Emergency Departments Treat 3.5 Million Crash Victims a Year," (January 13), 2010 [http://www.ahrq.gov/news/nn/nn011310.htm]

[11] Centers for Disease Control and Prevention, "Poisoning in the United States: Fact Sheet," (March 19, 2012) [http://www.cdc.gov/HomeandRecreationalSafety/Poisoning/poisoni ng-factsheet.htm] (Information collected after 2009 reports that accidental deaths related to prescription drug overdose have surpassed deaths caused by car accidents, see Chapter 11, footnote 9.

[12] Arbous, M., Grobbee, D., van Kleef, J., de Lange, J., Spoormans, H., Touw, P., Werner, F., Meursing, A., "Mortality Associated with

Anaesthesia: A Qualitative Analysis to Identify Risk Factors, (December 2001) *Anaesthesia*, Volume 56, Issue 12 pages 1141-1153

[13] Li, G., Warner, M., Lang, B., Huang, L., Sun, L., "Epidemiology of Anesthesia-related Mortality in the United States, 1999-2005," *Anesthesiology*, (April 2009) Volume 110, Issue 4 pages 759-765

[14] Baranov, D., Bickler, P., Crosby, G., Culley, D., Eckenhoff, M., "Consensus Statement: First International Workshop on Anesthetics and Alzheimer's Disease," (May 2009) *Anesthesia & Analgesia*, Volume 108, Issue 5 pages 1627-1630

[15] Health Affairs, The People-to-People Health Foundation, Anderson, G., Hussey, P., Frogner, B., Waters, H., "Health Spending in the United States and The Rest of the Industrialized World," (2012) [http://content.healthaffairs.org/content/24/4/903.full]

Chapter Twelve

Himmelstein, D., Thorne, D., Warren, E., Woolhandler, S., "Medical Bankruptcy in the United States, 2007: Results of a National Study" (2009) *The American Journal of Medicine*, Volume 122, Issue 8 pages 741-746

Made in the USA
Charleston, SC
25 July 2012